Reflections from Holland

A New Mother's Journey with Down Syndrome

Dana Hemminger

Reflections from Holland: A New Mother's Journey with Down Syndrome

Copyright © 2014 by Dana Hemminger

All rights reserved.

For additional copies, visit www.amazon.com

Scripture taken from the New King James Version ®. Copyright © 1982 by Thomas Nelson. Used by permission. All rights reserved.

Printed in the United States of America

ISBN-13: 978-1500269180

ISBN-10:1500269182

Dedication

First and foremost, I dedicate this book to my amazing God—Father, Son and Holy Spirit. Your constant love and tenderness has carried me through the most difficult days. In Your Presence there is truly joy in the midst of pain. I offer this book as worship unto You.

Next, I dedicate this to my wonderful husband Shawn and our little miracle Benjamin. I truly cherish our beautiful family!

Finally, I dedicate this to everyone who has ever loved a child with special needs. May the following pages offer you a measure of hope and healing as you walk out your own journey.

Table of Contents

Endorsements   1

Introduction   2

Part One: How Our Story Began…

    Company's Coming!   5
    Promise   12
    The Dream   14
    Unexpected Results   15
    It's a Boy! (Ultrasound Drama)   21
    It's Baby Day! (So soon???)   26
    Dashed Expectations   31
    A World Turned Upside-Down   35

Part Two: Grandma Jan's Journal

    A Special Poem   42
    How I Love Him Already! (May 2009)   43
    Grandma's Ramblings (June 2009)   51
    Best Picture   62
    A Note from Grandma Jan   63

Part Three: Stories and Reflections from a Mother's Heart

    "Broken"   66
    First Glimpse   68
    Projectile Poop!   72
    "Sighting Day"   74
    A Mended Heart   77
    Another Hurdle   84
    Joy in the Pain   91
    God's Formula   93
    Memories and Miracles   97
    Journey   98
    Sacrifice of Praise   103
    Eyes of the Beholder   106
    Touching Millions   110
    A Day at the Park   118
    Lessons from a Sippy Cup   122

To Wean or not to Wean?	127
Defining "Normal"	130
Embracing Change	134
Water Baby	137
The Power of Weakness	140
Someday	144
The Comparison Game	149
The Essence of Benjamin	153
Unconditional Love	164
True Value	166
Mr. Mobile	171
Help that Hurts	178
You Heard What I Said!	182
Treasures in Darkness	193
All I've Known is Holland	195
Step By Step	198
No More Excuses	203
A Time to Cherish	206
Dream Come True	211
About the Author	215

Endorsements

"(Y)our blog has been wonderful to read. It has given me a glimpse into your struggles and triumphs, sorrows and joys, and shown the overwhelming love and commitment you have for your family and God." – Marissa; elementary education paraprofessional

"You write so poetically, so honestly and so raw. I wanted to cry as I read about your day. You are such a strong, wise woman, and your words touched my heart with truth. Thank you." –Kassy; mother of child with special needs

"Wow, your faith is beautiful! I was literally in tears reading this story!...(Y)our have really encouraged me! Thanks for your transparency!" – Nicole; blog reader

"Thanks for sharing your heart so honestly…I have always been touched by the candid way you have expressed your feelings and experiences through your writing, and I know that many others have been blessed and will continue to be blessed as well." – Sharon; blog reader

"I have been wanting another child, but I am afraid of the same things…I don't ever want to find myself thinking or dwelling on how much quicker another child develops or learns. I want to enjoy every moment. Reading your story made me smile and made me believe that it will be ok whenever we embark on that new experience…Thank you! Your story is beautiful; keep telling it!" – Leeann; mother of child with Down syndrome

Introduction

Years ago a woman by the name of Emily Perl Kingsley wrote a beautiful essay entitled "Welcome to Holland" in order to express the unique experience of raising a child with a disability. She did a fantastic job of giving language to something that is often so difficult to articulate. Using allegory she describes pregnancy as preparing for a wonderful trip to Italy. You make so many plans and learn as much as you can while eagerly awaiting the big day. When it finally arrives you board the plane and touch down hours later only to hear the stewardess say "Welcome to Holland!" Amid the onslaught of shock and emotions you soon realize that your flight plan has been changed, and there is nothing you can do about it. Your dream of going to Italy is gone; meanwhile most of your friends continue to happily travel to Italy themselves. You realize that you must now learn a new language and culture for which you were not prepared. However, as you begin to get your bearings, you are able to realize that Holland has a beauty and grace all its own. Though there is pain that you did not make it to Italy, in time you are able to appreciate and enjoy your experiences in Holland.

This simple yet profound analogy straight from a mother's heart has given hope, encouragement, and perspective to countless parents and caregivers, myself included. On May 22, 2009, my husband and I began our own journey into Holland with the arrival of our first child, Benjamin Lee Hemminger. In our journey thus far we have experienced the greatest pain and the greatest joy we have ever known. Part of my healing process has been to write. At first the writing was only for myself and a few close loved ones. Near the beginning of 2011, a friend encouraged me to begin blogging and share our story with others. My blog, www.reflectionsfromholland.blogspot.com, became a treasured outlet to express my heart and to both give and receive encouragement. Near the end of 2011, through a series of events, I felt the Lord prompting me to begin collecting and compiling my writing into book form. Though the process has taken much longer than I anticipated, the result is what you now hold in your hands.

In the Psalms of the Old Testament, King David poured out his heart before the Lord with unhindered abandon. He expressed every emotion known to man. In the midst of it all, though, he clung to the Shepherd of his soul. This has been my story; clinging to Jesus only to realize He is holding me securely in His hands while I do my best to trust Him with each new step. In the following pages you will find a wide array of emotions. It has been my desire to write raw and real: to write the type of book I wish had been available to me when we began our journey. In some pages I re-tell parts of our story as though I were re-living the moment. In other pages I use written words to pour out my grief and pain. You will also find pages full of joy and celebration, as well as reflections on the lessons God has been teaching me thus far. I do not apologize for any of it. This is my heart, and this is my journey. Regardless of why you hold this book in your hands now, you are on your own unique journey as well, with your own experiences of joy and of pain. My prayer is that my story can bring you encouragement as you walk down the path of your own life. Thanks for reading…

Part One:

How Our Story Began…

Company's Coming!

There are two lines. Two pink lines. I stand in our tiny bathroom in stunned silence. Two lines—there have never been two lines. How many times have I rehearsed this moment in my mind during the last two years? I've lost count. I've pictured my reaction over and over. Will I scream? Jump up and down? Laugh? Cry? Instead, I stand in silence, studying the little strip again and again to make sure my eyes aren't playing tricks on me. After all the tears, all the disappointments, all the prayers, is the moment really here? I walk out of the bathroom in a daze where Shawn is anxiously waiting in the living room.

"Well?"

"There are two lines."

"What does that mean?"

"There have never been two lines."

The beautiful reality begins to sink in, and Shawn pulls me into a delighted embrace. The reality suddenly hits me like a wave as well, and the tears pour down. Deep, happy sobs erupt from the core of my being. We're going to have a baby!

I try to collect myself and call my mom, the only other person who knew I would be taking the test. She answers the phone to hear my sobs, and at first her heart sinks. Then through my tears I manage to blurt out. "Mom, we're going to have a baby! *(sob)* I'm really happy!"

Two years before, near the end of our first year of marriage, we were not trying to conceive—were even taking preventative measures—but my cycle was so late in coming. We finally decided to purchase a home pregnancy test. Shawn and I tried to be discreet in the store. We didn't want stories circling before anything was confirmed. Yet the more we thought about the possibility of pregnancy, the more excited we became. We held hands in the living room and prayed before I made my way back to the bathroom. My stomach was tied in knots of anticipation. I opened the test, read and re-read the instructions just to make sure. . . but I never used it. My cycle had just started. I cried all evening.

After that experience the birth control went out the window, and we were confident it wouldn't be long until I really did conceive. Yet the weeks turned into months, and the months began slipping into years and still no baby. Meanwhile, other young couples were conceiving, the wives aglow with bright smiles and beautiful rounded bellies. I wanted to be happy for them. I wanted to celebrate with them. I hated what I was feeling inside--jealousy, resentment, fear. *God, when will it be my turn?*

There were more false alarms. There were more tests actually taken only to show one line--one lousy pink line. I'd finally written off pregnancy tests. I wanted to throw them against the wall whenever I took one, only to be disappointed again. I promised myself I wouldn't consider another test until I was really, really sure.

******

The day before my test…

It's October 31, 2008. I sit with Shawn in the living room, sipping coffee before work. I log onto the laptop, open the Internet and search early pregnancy symptoms. As I read I realize I can check off almost every one.

"My cycle still hasn't started…I think it might be time to take a test again."

"Do you really think you might be pregnant this time?"

"I'm not sure what to think. I don't want to get my hopes up, but I have most of the early symptoms listed here. I'm so tired. I don't feel good. I have to pee constantly. My stomach's been cramping. And, my breasts are tender. They've never been tender before."

"Ok, we'll pick one up tomorrow."

I have tried so hard to find excuses for what I've been experiencing. I've been under stress. We've been busy at work. My immune system is just down right now. The tiredness is affecting my emotions. I've always had a fairly weak bladder. The cramps must mean my cycle will start any day now. I can't explain the tender breasts, though. This is a new experience.

The Salvation Army, where Shawn and I are both currently employed, is hosting a Fall Festival tonight to provide a safe and fun environment for families in the community. Shawn and I have also arranged to have a prayer room open for twelve hours, from noon to midnight in the sanctuary. We have encouraged people to sign up for one hour prayer slots. However, no one has signed up to pray and we are needed to work at the festival since it is a large undertaking. I'm tired, emotional, and I don't feel well. To make matters worse, a family that attends the Corps from time to time is there with their newborn daughter. *(In The Salvation Army the local church is referred to as the Corps)*. The baby's great-grandma sees me and hollers out, "When are you having one, Dana? We're all waiting for you!"

Outwardly I smile and say, "Whenever God decides to bless me." Inwardly I want to throw something at her. My nerves are raw. As if on cue, another woman from the Corps who has two teenage daughters and an eight year old son pulls me close and whispers in my ear, "We just found out I'm pregnant!"

I'm shocked. I feel like I've just been punched in the stomach. Again, outwardly I smile and hug her and congratulate her on the exciting news. Inwardly I want to melt into the floor. I just want to run away and have a good, long cry. *(My heart would break for her a few months later when she suffered a miscarriage. Her family kindly extended love and support to us throughout my pregnancy and during the shaky days that followed.)*

The night drags on and more reminders are thrown in my face. The wife of a co-worker, a young woman a few years younger than myself, is already blooming with their first child. She's wearing a hand-made tee-shirt with a jack-o-lantern on the front that fits just right around her growing abdomen. I can't stand how cute she looks. I can't stand that she was able to get pregnant so easily, while we've tried and tried. I can't stand the negative emotions I'm feeling towards people tonight. I don't want these ugly thoughts. A man with a camera targets us and wants to get a picture of the two young women. We stand together and pose. She smiles with her expectant glow; I plaster on a smile and hope to get away quickly.

The hotdogs I eat feel like rocks in my stomach. I don't ever want to see or smell a hotdog again. I'm so tired. Clean-up has finally begun. I pass Shawn in the gym. He's directing the workers and volunteers. I want to pour out my heart to him. I want him to hold me and tell me he loves me and that it's all going to be okay. Instead he distractedly hands me a push broom and asks me to sweep the gym floor. I should know better than to try to talk to him when he's focused on work. As I begin to clean I turn my heart to the Lord.

"God, my heart is hurting so much right now. I'm so afraid of being disappointed again."

I haven't forgotten you.

The phrase runs so clearly through my mind, and I am comforted. He sees me. He knows. My heart matters to Him.

Finally, it is time to go home. We will have about an hour to rest before returning to finish out the last two hours of the 12 hours of prayer—quite probably the only two hour slot that was filled. I share some of my thoughts and feelings with Shawn in the car.

"Honey, if you're too tired you can stay home. Get some rest. I'll go and pray."

I consider this before answering, "No, I want to come with you. I need to pray."

An hour later we step into the church sanctuary, which several hours before I had lovingly set up with specific prayer stations to encourage devotion and to give direction while praying. Bibles and journals are laid out. Huge sheets of paper hang on the walls with markers close by with which prayers can be written. Candles are waiting to be lit as a representation of each life prayed over. Water colors sit next to clear glasses of water, brushes ready to create colorful strokes and transform stark white paper into worshipful works of art. Silk flowers and greenery are delicately arranged; satin cloths cover the tables. Everything is so still; everything looks completely untouched. We've hosted successful prayer room events in the past, but this time everyone has been so busy. Feeling a new wave of discouragement hit me, I make my way to my personal favorite station—the quiet corner. An attractive wicker divider, silk trees, and plants enclose a far corner of the sanctuary. On the floor is a welcoming blanket. A lamp shines softly on a white pillar. I want to be alone with God right now, secluded from everything else, including my husband.

I sink to my knees and the tears begin to fall. Tonight was almost more than I could handle. I'm anxious for tomorrow's pregnancy test, wondering if I can take another disappointment if it turns out negative.

"Father, I need to hear from You. Please speak to my heart." I begin to write my thoughts and prayers in my journal.

"Read Psalm 68," the phrase runs softly through my mind.

I flip open my Bible and turn the thin pages to the Psalms. The 68th Psalm is rather long, 35 verses to be exact. The heading reads, "The Glory of God and His Goodness to Israel." I begin reading, wondering if I was hearing Him right. I resolve in my heart to read through the entire Psalm, though I'm beginning to doubt I was really hearing from God. I reach verse 27, and the words leap off the page *"There is little Benjamin, their leader..."* I read it again, amazed. Shawn and I have known all along that we would name our firstborn son Benjamin. We've also had a sense all along that our first child would be a boy. This verse seems so specific, yet I'm still afraid to hope too much. I write in my journal:

Thank You for reminding me tonight that You haven't forgotten me. Thank You that You understand all the emotions I'm experiencing even when it feels like nobody else does. Father, I ask that if I'm not pregnant that You would touch my body and cause my period to start tonight or in the morning. If I am pregnant, please let it be confirmed by the pregnancy test. Please cover my heart and Shawn's heart and prepare us for whatever the answer is right now. Thank You that Your timing is perfect and that You carefully direct our steps. I give this back to You, Abba, and I thank You that You always know best.

******

Now, the next morning, I'm sitting next to my husband on the couch, snuggled close as we make calls to family and a few close friends. The happy tears have given way to a peaceful calm, though it all still feels surreal in a joyful way. We call Shawn's dad and his older brother. We then call his mom and step-dad. Cyndi lets out a delighted scream at the news. The first grandbaby is coming. She's been saving a crib and changing table for ten years since Shawn's baby brother outgrew them. I smile thinking of my mother-in-law as a grandma. With her youthful appearance she's been mistaken as the girlfriend of her grown sons a time or two, a fact that appalls them both! A few more calls are made to grandparents and some out of town friends, but we decide to share in person with the rest of our local friends.

To celebrate we head back to the store and purchase the cute baby outfit I had my eye on earlier. It's a white and blue striped onesie with matching blue pants and a picture of a tan lion on the front. The lettering reads "L is for Lion who is loveable in every way." I've been planning for a long time to decorate Benjamin's nursery in lions. We also purchase two large pieces of fleece so I can make a baby blanket. The pattern I select has pictures of jungle animal babies, including lions. I pick a solid light green for the backing, and we happily move toward the check-out. As we make our purchase we see our friend Katie. I can't help myself; I have to tell her. She is thrilled and gives me a huge hug. I want to announce the good news to the entire store. I want to shout it from the rooftops. We're going to have a baby!

Promise

I'm in the first trimester of pregnancy. Some days it's hard to believe that my dream really has come true, and we are going to have a baby! The fleece I purchased to make a baby blanket has finally become a finished project. I started by cutting small strips around the borders of both pieces of fabric that could be tied together to form one thick blanket. I didn't have any instructions, but I figured I didn't really need them. How hard could it be? My first attempt resembled a circle more than a square; I'd tied the knots too tight. I untied them all and tried again. The second attempt was a little better but still not what I had pictured. I untied them again. (Not all in one sitting, mind you. My fingers were sore!) They say the third time's the charm, and in my case it was. I can't wait to wrap my baby in the blanket I lovingly prepared for him!

What will life look like with our baby, I wonder. What will he look like? What will his personality be? How will we adjust to being new parents? I have wanted this for so long! In the midst of my excitement, however, fear tries to rise and nag at my mind from time to time. I'm still so early in my pregnancy. What if something goes wrong? The thought of actually having a baby sometimes feels too good to be true. On one particular day, the worries have been rising in my heart. I know that worry is never from Jesus, so I sit down with Bible in hand, tell Him my fears, pray for our baby, and ask Him to speak to me. Psalm 71 comes to my mind, so I turn there and begin to read. As I read verse 5-6, tears of gratitude begin to flow:

For You are my hope, O Lord God; You are my trust from my youth. By You I have been upheld from birth; You are He who took me out of my mother's womb. My praise shall be continually of You.

There is a footnote in my Bible for the word *upheld* that reads *sustained from the womb*. I am so encouraged! He so quickly spoke to me, offering me peace to replace my fears. I journal this experience and share it with Shawn, who is encouraged as well. I don't know it now, but this word will become my prayer for Benjamin throughout the pregnancy. This word will become an anchor for my heart in the days and weeks following his birth. This word will become the promise I cling to time and again on the darkest of days. Sometimes all you have to hold on to is the word of God.

The Dream

November 23, 2008: I had a vivid dream last night…

I was lying on a hospital bed getting ready to have an ultrasound with Shawn by my side. I looked expectantly up at the screen, eager to catch a glimpse of my baby. Instead, the blank screen suddenly took the form of ancient parchment paper, and I witnessed the hand of God begin to write things concerning my unborn son. He began by saying "This is Benjamin." I couldn't remember what specific things He wrote about Benjamin's life, but the message was clear. "He will be okay, and I have good plans for him." Shawn and I were thrilled! Just as suddenly as the parchment appeared on the screen, it vanished, and a small boy whom we did not know appeared in the room and began to taunt us by saying of our son "His name is Saul! His name is Saul!" A righteous indignation rose within me, and I looked at him square in the eye. With authority in my voice I addressed the boy, "His name is Benjamin, and you will call him Benjamin!" The boy fell silent and I looked back at to the ultrasound screen where my baby now came into view. I saw an almost full-term infant, writhing inside my womb in obvious distress.

Before I had time to respond I awoke. After discussing it with Shawn, I jot down this intriguing dream in my journal and continue to write: *We wonder if God is preparing our hearts that there may be complications, but everything will turn out all right.*

Surely everything will be okay…

Unexpected Results

January 7, 2009:

I'm a few weeks into my second trimester. The queasiness of the first trimester has disappeared, and the early fatigue is beginning to lessen. I feel so relieved that I never experienced full blown morning sickness. I'm delighted with my growing "baby bump," and I'm enjoying my new wardrobe of maternity clothes. The faint flutters I occasionally feel in my womb are thrilling evidence of the life growing inside of me. I love being pregnant!

I have an appointment scheduled with my obstetrician, Dr. Cook, today, and I can't wait for another chance to hear our baby's heartbeat. I'm disappointed when I find out the nurse will be drawing more blood today. I've never liked needles (who does?), but I remind myself it's for the baby. The anticipated joy of our coming child is worth all necessary discomfort. After the nurse draws my blood, Dr. Cook explains to Shawn and me that this is a quad-screen test, which checks for potential birth defects or genetic abnormalities. I politely listen as he explains the details, though I am confident that none of this could possibly apply to us. He explains that an abnormal result on this blood test does not *diagnose* a condition, but rather verifies the increased *likelihood* of a possible condition. For curiosity sake, I ask what would be done in the case of an abnormal test result. He mentions amniocentesis or specialized ultrasounds as the means for obtaining an actual diagnosis, though amniocentesis is the most accurate. I tell him that I would not be comfortable with an amniocentesis because of the small yet potential risk of miscarriage connected with the procedure. He already knows our stance on abortion; nothing could ever convince us to take our baby's life. I feel a bit funny that we are even having this discussion. I know that our baby will be healthy and whole, and I don't see much use in discussing the "what-ifs?" Dr. Cook assures us that if for any reason my test comes back abnormal, he will call us personally; otherwise, he will discuss my test with me at the following visit. "I know everything will be fine," I say, and he smiles as we wrap up the appointment. Though I don't feel like all the information was necessary, I am thankful for a doctor who takes the time to explain things to us.

******

January 12, 2009:

I am sitting at my desk at The Salvation Army where I am employed as an overseer for the small Christian Education department. While working, I chat on and off with my friend and co-worker Mandy who shares the office with me. We are interrupted when my cell phone rings.

"Hello?"

"Dana, this is Dr. Cook."

I feel like my heart stops beating. There's only one reason he would be calling me this week.

"I'm sorry to tell you that while most of your test results came back normal, there was a positive result that you run a heightened risk of carrying a child with Down syndrome."

How do I begin to process what he's saying? I feel so numb.

Dr. Cook gently goes on to explain that a woman my age (26) typically runs a risk rate of 1 in 956 to give birth to a child with Down syndrome. My test results increase my risk factor to 1 in 270. He says he will refer me to a specialist to schedule an ultrasound in which they will measure my baby's bone growth and look for any "markers" for Down syndrome. He assures me again that the blood test is not diagnostic and often further testing yields normal results. He encourages me that I can feel free to call if I have any additional questions and that I should be expecting to hear from the specialist soon. Fighting to contain my composure, I thank Dr. Cook for calling and hang up the phone.

"Is everything okay?" Mandy inquires. Her face is full of concern from what little she heard from my end of the conversation. I'm sure my expression gives it away as well. With a shaky voice I relay back to her my conversation with the doctor, saying periodically to comfort myself, "I'm sure everything will turn out okay." My friend doesn't know what to say and tries her best to offer some word of encouragement. I quickly excuse myself to go find Shawn.

I find my husband at the other end of the building, alone with his laptop and a book. The moment I walk into the room he asks, "What's wrong?" The tears begin to flow as I blurt out with a sob, "Everything's going to be okay!" It hurts me to tell him, knowing the pain he will feel as well. We sit together in shock, silent tears running down our faces. How could this possibly be happening? We have wanted a baby for so long. We pray over my womb every day. We envision the perfect, healthy baby boy scheduled to arrive in the summer. Surely the test is wrong!

We make our way up to Captain Gargis' office. He is our current supervisor and pastor, but he and his family will soon be transferred to another Salvation Army Corps. *(The Salvation Army uses military terms to address clergy, and church members are referred to as soldiers)*. Over the last year and half, he has mentored us in his fatherly way, and he has always willingly offered a listening ear. In his wisdom, he doesn't try to find a quick answer to make us feel better. He listens to us, cries with us, and shares in our shock and pain. He assures us of the love we will have for our child regardless of his or her condition and takes the time to pray with us. He also gives us the option of taking the afternoon off so that we can have some time to process the news we just received. Shawn tells me he will take an extended lunch break with me, but he will have to return in the afternoon to assist with school pick-ups for the after school program he directs. He will come home again as soon as he can get away.

Our drive home is marked by tears and prayers, but surprisingly, by the time we pull into our driveway, an unexpected peace has descended on our hearts, and we know others are praying for us. Once inside I quickly grab my pregnancy book to see if there is any information on Down syndrome and the testing I just received. As Shawn and I read about some of the common traits of a child with Down syndrome, it feels so surreal to think that this could be our child. We don't feel at all ready to accept that reality and are encouraged to read that things such as a miscalculated due date or even the presence of twins can result in a false-positive reading. Surely this is the case with us. As I take time to read and pray, I receive strength from Psalm 138:3, 7-8….

In the day when I cried out, You answered me, and made me bold with strength in my soul…Though I walk in the midst of trouble, You will revive me; You will stretch out Your hand against the wrath of my enemies, and Your right hand will save me. The Lord will perfect that which concerns me; Your mercy, O Lord, endures forever. Do not forsake the work of Your hands.

After supper we head out to meet up with some friends from Nightwatch, a weekly prayer and worship gathering we have been a part of for the last four to five years. Tonight we will be carpooling to a neighboring town where a church is hosting a minister named Bobby Conner. On the way Shawn and I ask the Lord to speak to us specifically tonight about our unborn baby.

The service is good, but it's hard to fully focus with this unanswered question hanging over my head. There is still a peace guarding my heart, but there is the presence of pain as well. Near the end, Mr. Conner is walking through the congregation, quietly asking the Holy Spirit to highlight people to him and give him words of encouragement to share with them. As he does this, he continues to preach some and tell stories. He is a delight to listen to—very funny at times, but when he speaks, our hearts are so stirred for Jesus. The Word of God continually flows out from him because he has taken the time to really get it inside of him. As a result, he walks very closely with the Lord and hears His voice. When he is close to our section, I silently pray again, "Lord, please speak to us tonight about our baby." Within moments, he stops in front of Shawn and me and begins to engage us briefly in conversation. He then points to my pregnant belly and declares, "I speak John the Baptist over your baby. He will be full of the Holy Spirit from the womb." *(Incidentally, this same thing was spoken over Benjamin on three more occasions during my pregnancy by three different ministers, none of whom were connected to one another!)*

Shawn and I are thrilled! John the Baptist was born in seemingly impossible circumstances and was set apart for God before he was even conceived. He walked closely with God and prepared the way for an entire generation to recognize and receive Jesus when He came. How exciting to think that our baby will be one set apart from the womb, whose life will prepare the way for many to meet Jesus!

More encouragement comes before the night is over. A layman in the church is a close friend to Mr. Conner and has travelled with him before. He is invited up at the end to share anything that he feels the Holy Spirit has been speaking to him. Without hesitation he points me out of the crowd and says, "I'm supposed to tell you that God is going to put a lot of vitamins and nutrients in your blood, making it rich with iron." I almost fall out of my chair! This feels so incredibly personal after lamenting all day over my abnormal *blood* test! He shares words of encouragement with two more people and then asks for Shawn and me to come over to where he and his wife are so that they can pray for us. We tell them all about the test and the call that day. They encourage us, pray for us, and promise to be praying for us regularly. He asks us to bring the baby back to meet them after he's born. Our hearts are soaring!

Before leaving, we purchase a book from Mr. Conner and ask him to sign it. He does so and jots down the scripture reference Isaiah 44:3-4…

For I will pour water on him who is thirsty, and floods on the dry ground; I will pour My Spirit on your descendents, and My blessing on your offspring; They will spring up among the grass like willows by the watercourses.

We feel like we are floating out of the church. With so much personal encouragement tonight, how could our baby possibly have Down syndrome?

It's a Boy! (Ultrasound Drama)

January 16, 2009:

Shawn and I sit in a large waiting room at St. John's Hospital in Tulsa, Oklahoma, waiting for my appointment with Dr. Blake, the specialist who will conduct the ultrasounds for our unborn baby. After what feels like an extremely long wait, we are escorted back to a small room. I am instructed to lie on the examination table and Shawn takes a seat in the corner. We notice a flat screen monitor attached to the wall, easily viewable from both of our vantage points. A young woman steps in and explains that she is one of the technicians who will be conducting most of the ultrasound; Dr. Blake will take a look at the end and visit with us.

We are both so eager. The only ultrasound I've had so far was at the very beginning of my pregnancy. At that point our baby looked like a peanut-sized blob on the screen, but his heart was already beating! We can't wait to see what our child will look like at 17 weeks gestation and hope that the little boy we believe him to be will be clearly identified! We are slightly anxious about what the ultrasound will reveal, though we feel mostly confident that the quad-screen test was a false-positive for Down syndrome.

The technician has me lift my shirt over my rounded belly and smears a warm, clear goop all over. She then takes the ultrasound wand and starts to move it slowly across my baby bump. A picture appears on the screen, but at first it's hard to make out what we are seeing. She is very accommodating, answering our questions and identifying for us what we are viewing on the monitor. She explains that the ultrasound will take awhile, as she must take detailed measurements of every part of our baby. I appreciate how she always refers to him as "baby," not "it," or "fetus," or some other sterile word. This is our child, and his life is precious.

We are thrilled by some of the images we see. Our little guy is so active, swimming all around in Mommy's womb. We recognize a side shot of his head and are captured by his profile. He lifts a tiny fist up to his mouth as though he's getting ready to suck! We see an arm; we see a leg; we see many things we can't readily identify. We are awestruck that we are actually watching our baby move around inside my body. He's really there, and he's really coming! He also seems to prefer to tuck his head down into my right side, making it difficult for the technician to get some of the measurements she needs. She has me take a bathroom break, hoping my movement will cause him to move as well. Once back, we ask her if she can determine our baby's sex or not. Seemingly on cue, Benjamin spreads his legs wide, as if to proudly declare, "I am Benjamin, and there's no mistaking it!" We really are having a boy!

We notice that the technician keeps going back to look at his heart. She says that she's having a hard time seeing all that she needs to see. We think nothing of it and are excited the ultrasound is lasting a bit longer. After awhile she explains that she will need to ask Dr. Blake to get those parts of the measurements; she's not been successful in obtaining them. She graciously excuses herself and tells us the doctor will be with us shortly.

Shawn and I are so excited. The technician printed some pictures for us before leaving, and we can't wait to get back to work and show them off! Benjamin is Benjamin! A few minutes later Dr. Blake steps in. We can tell from the beginning that she's not going to be one for much conversation but is there to professionally accomplish the task at hand and then move on to the next one as efficiently as possible. She also takes some extra time examining our son's heart, but we figure it must be difficult to measure something so small, especially when the baby's so active. When she finally completes the ultrasound, she explains, much to our relief, that our baby's measurements look normal. She does not see any obvious markers for Down syndrome. He weighs a whopping 7 oz., and his heart is beating at 123 beats per minute—all within normal range. She says she would like to schedule two more ultrasounds, six weeks apart, just to keep an eye on his development. We are a little surprised by this, but the thought of seeing our baby two more times before he is born is exciting! We witnessed a miracle today. How could anyone deny that the active little life inside of me is a baby? His life is so valuable!

******

May 8, 2009:

It's raining cats and dogs this morning. We are scheduled to see Dr. Blake again in a few hours for our last of the three ultrasounds. The second one in March was less dramatic than the first. Since Benjamin had grown (as he should), it was very difficult to identify anything we were seeing on the screen, which was a bit disappointing. His measurements still looked normal, and we were sent on our way. Today, I don't really want to go. My body has gone through drastic change, even within the last month. My belly is huge! I'm carrying Benjamin all out front and low. My ankles and feet are swollen, and I can't walk without waddling. I'm exhausted from broken sleep every night. I can no longer sleep on my side and instead sleep in the living room recliner. I say "sleep," but it's more like a series of short naps throughout the night. Benjamin is moving like crazy, and though I love seeing and feeling him move, some of his activity has become painful. We are already driving to Owasso, forty minutes away, on a weekly basis at this point to see Dr. Cook. The thought of an hour drive to Tulsa this morning is not appealing. Everything has been fine so far, and while it would be neat to see the ultrasound (maybe), I wonder if it's worth all the energy it will take. "Lord, if you want us to go, please let it stop raining. If not, I'm going to call and cancel."

It stops raining. Somewhat reluctantly, we load up in the car for the long drive. We are so blessed to have another pair of understanding supervisors, who not only allow for me to take time off for my multiple appointments, but who also allow my husband to accompany me. Captains Carlyle and Charlotte Gargis were transferred in January, and Majors Alan and Cheryl Phillips arrived from Florida shortly thereafter. We miss the Gargis family, but we also enjoy building relationship with the Majors. They are very supportive of my pregnancy. I'm thankful as well for Shawn's willingness to come with me, especially now that it's getting more difficult for me to drive, but I know he is getting a bit weary as well…

As we expected, it is very difficult to identify what we are seeing on the ultrasound screen unless someone explains it to us. Benjamin is just too big at this point. The abundance of amniotic fluid around him in the first ultrasound provided the perfect backdrop to distinguish his movements and features. He takes up most of the space now, and only a trained eye can recognize anything at all. As usual, Dr. Blake takes a few moments to discuss the ultrasound with us. Our baby's measurements still look good, though his belly measures two weeks bigger than the rest of him. It looks like I'm carrying a little chunk! We are startled, however, when she informs us that my amniotic fluid is measuring low. What does that mean? How does that happen? She explains that there's not a clear reason why it happens, but if my levels drop too low, our baby can be in danger of settling on top of the umbilical cord and pinching off the flow of oxygen and nutrients to his body. If my amniotic fluid drops below a certain level, it will require an emergency delivery. My levels are not to the danger point yet, but they are not good. She wants to see us back weekly until the baby is born to conduct both a non-stress test and an ultrasound. Our hearts sink. We have five weeks to go until my due date. How can we keep up with this pace?!

May 13, 2009

I have my weekly appointment with Dr. Cook, and he explains that, due to my low fluid, there's no way I will go all the way to my due date. He will have to induce labor early, though he hopes to get me to 37 weeks. That's only three weeks away! I've heard that induced labors tend to be more difficult. This is not how I wanted things to go!

Later in the day I call our trusted friend, Myong, an amazing woman from South Korea who has been a spiritual mother to us for the last few years. I tearfully tell her about the doctor's report. I'm not sure what to think or feel. I know our baby will be okay, but I'm scared, too. Today's news was so unexpected, and I'm exhausted, which is only heightening my emotions. She prays with me on the phone, and she is fired up. She's going to fight in prayer for our baby's well-being. She encourages me that Shawn's and my prayers for our son are so important and so powerful. She encourages me to worship through this; it will be life to me and life to our baby. I place my hand on my stomach and silently pray over my son. I am comforted by his movement. I remind myself of the many promises spoken over him throughout my pregnancy. He is going to be okay.

It's Baby Day! (So Soon?)

May 15, 2009:

We are at St. John's Hospital again for the first of our now weekly appointments with Dr. Blake. A nurse leads us back to a small room and instructs me to lie back on the hospital table as she makes the necessary preparations for the non-stress test. Benjamin's only been slightly active this morning, so I hope he will cooperate. The nurse straps a few circular, palm-size monitors over my bulging belly, putting pressure on my womb. She explains that I will need to lie still for the next 20-30 minutes as the monitors track our baby's movement and heartbeat. A machine close by will be printing out the results throughout the duration of the test. She tells me to relax and leaves Shawn and me alone in the room, saying she will be back to check on us and on the results periodically.

As soon as the monitors are in place, my inactive little boy suddenly becomes very active! He does not appreciate the extra pressure on his little abode. Shawn and I watch with amusement (and I with some discomfort as well) as our baby attempts with all his might to kick off the offending monitors! I have never seen my stomach move like this—waves would really be the best description! When the test is finally complete, the nurse unhooks me and explains that the results look good today. (We were sure they would.) She then leads us to another room where I will have an ultrasound to complete part two of today's testing. Benjamin obviously wore himself out during the non-stress test, and he doesn't move much as measurements are taken of my amniotic fluid levels. He must be napping. We are relieved to learn that my fluid has actually gone up slightly since last week!

May 18, 2009:

We're once again sitting in Dr. Cook's office for my weekly check-up. We will be seeing Dr. Blake again at the end of the week. However, he believes that next week's appointment with her will be the real determining factor for when he will induce labor. He explains that he will be leaving town this weekend for the Memorial Day holiday. While it's unlikely that I will need to be induced this weekend, he wants us to understand that in the event something should happen, I will be attended to by one of the doctors on call.

"It's probably not going to happen," he says, concluding his thoughts. We agree. We do follow the recommendation, however, to have a hospital bag packed in the car, "just in case."

******

May 19, 2009:

Shawn and I sit in a conference room at Jane Phillips Medical Center in Bartlesville for our third of four childbirth classes. I am so looking forward to the end of the class tonight when all the dads get to take a turn wearing the "sympathy belly." When the time comes, each man dutifully straps on the thirty-pound vest, complete with a bulging belly and breasts, and he must bend down to pick up a pencil on the floor. The room is full of laughter and flashing cameras. Shawn and I have our picture taken together when it's his turn, but my belly definitely has his beat! His five minutes of baby belly weight is nothing compared to my past few months of constant kicks, sleepless nights and a squashed bladder! Next week's class, when we will learn about breastfeeding, is the one I'm looking forward to the most. I've dreamed all my life of nursing my babies, and I can't wait for that special bond! As an eighteen-month-old nursing child myself, I stood up solemnly in the middle of church one Sunday evening, lifted my dress over my shoulder, and pressed my baby doll's face up to my baby chest. I guess I've looked forward to this for a long time!

******

May 20, 2009:

It's a warm day with summer just around the corner. I'm wearing a one piece cotton dress and my newly purchased Croc sandals--the only shoes my hot, swollen feet can handle at this point. I've wrapped up most of my Christian Education responsibilities at The Salvation Army. All that remains now is to clean out my office space and assist in Social Services as I'm able to until it's time to deliver the baby. My desk is almost cleaned off, but I still have to tackle the bookcase. Sitting on the floor is going to be necessary to clean out and organize the bottom shelves. Getting down isn't so bad; getting up, however, is another story! I'm so glad Mandy's close by. What will it be like to be able to do simple tasks like bending over again? It feels like a lifetime ago since I was able to do that. Some days it's hard to remember what it was like to *not* be pregnant...

...Since it is Wednesday night, Shawn and I are leading the youth group meeting at The Salvation Army. Tonight we are talking about trusting God. Our current situation creates the perfect illustration:

"We really have to trust God right now. It's possible that when I go to see the specialist tomorrow, she will tell me that I can't go home and must be admitted to the hospital to deliver the baby. We have a bag packed in the car just in case." (Of course, we have little expectation that this will actually happen.)

We go on to share that part of trusting God is being totally honest with Him. When we're going through stuff, it's good to share with

Him all the rawness of our emotions. He's big enough to handle it, and He loves our honesty. We encourage the teens to pour their hearts out to God about any and every situation they face. He will meet them there.

******

May 21, 2009:

Benjamin has hardly moved this morning. As we make the drive to Tulsa, I talk to him and pray over him. "Come on, baby. You need to wake up and be active so they can monitor you." Surely he'll get going again once they strap those intruding monitors in place…

He must really be sleepy this morning. Even with the monitors strapped down, he's not doing a whole lot today. There's some movement here and there, but nothing like the waves we saw last week. Surely it's nothing to worry about…

The nurse keeps coming in and out to read the results as they print. She even brings some other nurses with her. No one is saying anything to us, but this doesn't feel like a normal silence. Soon I'm being unstrapped, and the nurse says we'll be going to speak with Dr. Blake now.

"…to do the ultrasound?" I inquire.

"I don't think there will be an ultrasound today," she replies.

Shawn and I sit in another room waiting for the doctor to come and tell us what in the world is going on. We are both feeling very uneasy, and we are trying hard not to jump to any conclusions. When Dr. Blake finally walks in, she exclaims "Well, it looks like it's baby day!" We just look at her in shock, trying to process what she has just said. Our minds swim as she explains that Benjamin's heart rate dropped for over a minute during the non-stress test.

While it's back up again, she feels that it would be in his best interest to deliver him now at 35 weeks. Otherwise, I would have to remain hospitalized and monitored 24/7 for the next few weeks to ensure his well-being. If his heart rate dropped once, it could do it again. It's possible that this has already been happening.

Dr. Blake instructs us to head down the road to Hillcrest Medical Center, where Dr. Cook happens to be practicing that day. We've never even seen the facility. We were planning to deliver at St. John's Hospital in Owasso. In a daze we check out at the front desk and head to the car. I am so grateful now that we had the presence of mind to pack a bag, though it's a fairly meager one. As Shawn drives I call my mom and tearfully give her the update, requesting that she fly out as soon as possible. My heart sinks as I realize that she won't be able to be with me during labor after all. I had pictured her and Shawn and possibly Myong staying with me through labor. They all bring such a calming presence. I'm so scared. This is all happening too fast. We knew this was a possibility, but I feel so unprepared. The nursery isn't finished yet. Shawn was going to finish painting the dresser this weekend, and we were going to get everything arranged just right for Benjamin. How can this be happening?!

Dashed Expectations

We pull into Hillcrest Medical Center and Shawn finds a place to park. I feel as though I'm walking through a dream as we find the correct entrance and get directions for check-in at the front desk. This is so surreal. Am I really having my baby today? As I begin speaking with an intake staff member to fill out the necessary paper work, I tearfully explain, "I'm having a baby today." The woman assisting me seems surprised by my response; having a baby is a happy thing! Everything just feels too sudden, too soon, and I'm concerned for Benjamin. I'm so anxious to get hooked up to a monitor again so I can know that he's doing okay. Finally, we are escorted up to a room.

A talkative, middle-aged nurse is in the room to get things started. She instructs me to take out my contacts, undress and get into a hospital gown. She will then get me hooked up with an IV line and fetal monitoring. I do things as quickly as possible, feeling as though every second could count for my son's well-being. I remind myself that things must not be too dangerous or else Dr. Blake would have admitted me right then and there, instead of sending us to another hospital. I wince as the IV line is inserted, but I have to laugh at myself with the reluctant realization that the sting of a needle is nothing compared to the labor pain I'm about to face. I want to do things naturally if possible, but I have not ruled out the option of having an epidural either.

Meanwhile, Shawn sits on the built-in couch, eating his portion of the lunch we packed. I was so emotional in the car, eating was the last thing on my mind. However, now that I'm hooked up to my IV and will be receiving Pitocin soon to induce labor, I am not allowed to eat or drink. I wish I had the presence of mind to eat while we were on the way. I had a bowl of oatmeal this morning and a banana in the car on the way to Tulsa, but I feel the hunger pains starting, and who knows at this point when I'll be allowed to eat again. Shawn is a ball of nervous, excited energy. He keeps saying, "We're going to have our baby today! We get to meet him!" I know I should feel excited, but I'm so nervous about labor and delivery, and I'm still in shock from the suddenness of everything.

Dr. Cook walks in with a sympathetic look on his face, and I'm so relieved to see him! Thankfully he is not scheduled to leave until sometime tomorrow. I'm so glad he will be the one to deliver Benjamin and not a stranger. He checks to see if I'm dilated at all so far, but I'm only at a two. My body wasn't planning on having a baby today. He explains that the nurse will get the Pitocin started, increasing or decreasing the amount I receive as necessary. He will be back to check on me periodically to measure how far I've dilated. It's really happening!

While I wait for the Pitocin to kick in, some friends from Bartlesville arrive, Myong being one. I am thankful to see them. They pray for me and the baby. So far Benjamin is doing very well. He's active off and on, and the fetal monitoring does not show anything that would cause alarm. I wonder how long it will take until contractions begin…

A few hours into receiving Pitocin, I begin to notice the first contraction. It doesn't hurt; it's just slightly uncomfortable. I focus on relaxed breathing and soon it's over. Every so often another one begins, and I close my eyes and breathe and pray. I soon lose all track of time and drift in and out of sleep. One friend tries to dialogue with me, but as the contractions begin to increase bit by bit, talking takes too much energy. They hurt some, but the pain is tolerable. How long will my labor be, I wonder?..

It's time to check my dilation again. I'm disappointed to find out I'm only at a three. This could be a much longer process than I hoped. It's dinner time, and our friends go to get some food and bring some back for Shawn. I wish I could eat. I'm so hungry and so tired. I try to focus on how wonderful it will be to hold Benjamin. He'll be in my arms soon enough!..

It's evening time, and I've only dilated to a four. The contractions are consistent but still not intense. Dr. Cook mentions the possibility of a C-section if my body doesn't begin to progress, but because Benjamin is doing well, I still have complete freedom to decide to keep trying for a natural delivery. As the evening presses on, Dr. Cook lets me know that he will be going home to rest, but he is on call and able to come back at a moment's notice if necessary. The nursing staff will keep an eye on my progress and will keep him updated as need be. If he does not hear from them sooner, he will be back early in the morning to attend to me. I had so hoped Benjamin would already be here by now.

******

May 22, 2009:

The hours plod on, but my body is not cooperating. I do not want to have a C-section, but as the night drags on, and my energy drains, I wonder how much longer I can go. I pray, "Lord, give me wisdom. What would be the best for Benjamin?" The fetal monitoring continues to show him in stable condition. I can no longer sleep due to the contractions, but I try to rest between each one as best as I can. Shawn has finally collapsed on the couch, and I envy his sleep…

It's 4:00 am, and I'm still only dilated to a four after over thirteen hours on Pitocin. I wake Shawn up and tell him with a tremor in my voice that I am considering a C-section. He's surprised but will be supportive of whatever decision I make. Resigned to this unwelcome course of action, I communicate to the nurse that I am too tired to go on at this pace. She contacts Dr. Cook, who quickly arrives to prepare me for my C-section. I visit with him and with the anesthesiologist and sign the necessary paperwork, indicating that I am aware of the risks involved with having a spinal and with the surgery. Is this really happening to me? My mind is so foggy from lack of food and sleep. I'm so tired, but now fear is beginning to set in as well. I've never had a surgery, never had a broken bone, and never even had stitches! In fact, this is my first time in a hospital. (My brother and I were both born at home.)

As I sit on the side of the hospital bed, signing papers and getting ready to be led down to the surgery room, my hands and arms begin to shake. Is this from the fear? Is this from the medicine? I am disturbed that I can't seem to control my own limbs. I hear a woman screaming from another delivery room down the hall. Dr. Cook tries to give me a reassuring smile, letting me know it won't be "that bad." But what will it be? The last fifteen hours feel like a bad dream. Nothing is as I expected.

A World Turned Upside Down

I waddle down the long hallway, IV lines in tow as though I'm floating through a dream. Shawn walks beside me, holding my hand until the inevitable parting outside the surgery room, a separation that happens all too quickly. He is directed to the recovery area where he must stay put while the pre-operation preparations are completed. Everything inside me is screaming for him to come with me, but I remain silent. I feel so scared, so alone. My body continues to shake. The young brunette nurse gently leads me into the operating room where I'm seemingly transported into another world. Everything is stark white; the lights are so bright I wish I had a pair of sunglasses; and it's cold, unbelievably cold. I'm told to sit on the operating table, so close to the edge I'm sure I'll fall off any moment, and slouch down low, as my spine is exposed through the back of the hospital gown. The shaking increases, and again I wonder if this is from the effects of the medicine, the cold, or the fear. Perhaps it's all three, but hard as I try, I cannot stop shaking. Horrible thoughts race through my mind. What if the shaking causes the spinal to go wrong? What if I'm paralyzed? Oh, Lord, please help me to stop shaking. I wish Shawn was here.

The brunette nurse puts her arms firmly but gently on my shoulders and lets me lean into her as the anesthesiologist rubs sterilizing solution over my back. The nurse is younger than I, but right now she feels like a mother. Right now she is my only tangible form of comfort, of stability. The anesthesiologist tells me I will feel a poke that may hurt, but it will not last long. I brace myself, feeling all the while like a frightened little girl. I just want to run away, reverse the clock even 24 hours when I still had the hopes of a close to full-term pregnancy and a natural labor and delivery. It's all happening too fast, too soon. I feel the jab, and it's painful. An apology, I'll have to be poked again. This time it hurts more, and always, the constant shaking. Within moments a warm, tingling sensation surges through my legs, and I am relieved to have some respite from the extreme cold. The next thing I know I'm being picked up and placed flat on my back, but I feel nothing from the waist down. I'm aware that my hospital gown is being lifted up above my waist—full exposure in a room of men and women, all wearing blue scrubs and face masks. I'm tempted to feel embarrassed, but all the other emotions quickly push down any concern for modesty or dignity—exhaustion, shock, fear, anticipation. I'll see my baby soon. Just a little while, I tell myself, and Benjamin will be in arms. Meanwhile the oxygen mask is being fitted over my nose and mouth, and the huge blue sheet is hung up in front of me. My husband appears by my head now, and relief washes over me. He tells me he loves me; I'm doing a good job; and everything will be okay. We're having our baby! He even snaps a picture.

The shaking has intensified as the spinal fully sets in. My arms seem to have a complete mind of their own, and move constantly on both sides of me, causing my voice to shake when I speak. Now a new fear sets in. Will the spinal be fully effective? What if I feel the cut? I brace myself, wondering when it will come. The next thing I know I feel a pulling and pushing on my stomach (no pain), and my son's first cry cuts through the cold, sterile air. My son, my baby I've been anticipating for so long: that is his cry. He's actually arrived! I try to contain my excitement as I wait for him to be cleaned up and brought over so I can see him. Shawn watches the doctor pull him out of my stomach and exclaims "He's so long!" He excuses himself from me for a minute to go snap pictures while Benjamin is being cleaned up. I hear my newborn's cries becoming more and more distant. Meanwhile, I feel a slight pulling while my stomach is stapled shut. How thankful I am for the blue sheet that shields my eyes from the gruesome process. I remember the video of a C-section in one of our childbirth classes.

In the car on the way home I cried and told Shawn "I don't want to have a C-section."

"Why would you have to have a C-section?" he asks.

"I don't know," I reply, "but I don't want to have one."

Now my impatience is starting to grow. Why is it taking so long for the nurses to clean up my baby? I want to see him. I start asking if they are going to bring him to me soon, but no one is answering me. Shawn reappears, his face full of concern. My head is swimming as he tells me that Benjamin is having some breathing problems. They're taking him down to the NICU to hook him up to a ventilator and do some more monitoring. I'm trying to process what he just said, but my mind is too fuzzy from all of the medicine, and my body is exhausted. I'm still shaking. I'm lifted from the operation table and placed on a hospital bed, then wheeled into the recovery area.

Shawn is given a chair next to my bed. I waste no time in asking him to show me the pictures he took of Benjamin. A picture is better than nothing, and I'm aching to see what my baby looks like. From the first picture, I know. I know, but I don't want to admit to myself that I know. I hear myself ask Shawn, "What's wrong with his neck?" It's so thick, almost like his head is set directly on top of a pair of shoulders with a thick crease of skin in the back. I ask again, "What's wrong with his neck?" Shawn just looks at me and says nothing. He knows it, too. He saw it as the nurses were cleaning up our son. Neither of us can bring ourselves to say the words that are hanging so heavy in the air, suffocating us. Benjamin looks like he has Down syndrome. I look at the pictures again and again, as though they might change if I keep studying them long enough. This can't be my baby. This isn't what I imagined he'd look like. There must be some mistake. I long for some words of comfort, some reassurance that this is all a bad dream from which I will wake at any moment. The effects of the medicine are too much for my exhausted system and I drift in and out of a fitful sleep. Shawn leans his head against the wall and does the same. All we can do is wait…

Dr. Jackson is by my bedside. She's a professional African-American woman with short-cut hair and beautiful but serious eyes. In a clear and steady voice she tells us that Benjamin is having significant trouble breathing and is hooked up to a ventilator, which is doing most of his breathing for him. She also tells us that she has ordered a genetic test because Benjamin has some physical characteristics of Down syndrome. There, the dreaded words have been spoken. Our hopes that we were somehow mistaken are dashed to pieces. She has more to say, but I can't take it in right now. My world is spinning out of control, even as my body has been for the last few hours, shaking, shaking, shaking. I ask again when I can see my baby, but I'm given no definite answers. Everything is out of control…

It's been over an hour and still I have no feeling from the waist down. The anesthesiologist said that the effects of the spinal usually begin to wear off in an hour. What if my fears are coming true? What if I'm paralyzed? After the shock and trauma of the doctor's news, this almost seems inevitable. Everything is already going horribly wrong. A nurse comes in to pinch my toes and poke my legs. "Any feeling?" she asks.

"Nothing," I reply

"Can you try to move your toes?"

I muster up all the strength I have into focusing on moving just one toe, but it seems useless. I can't feel a thing. The fear is mounting. My upper body is still shaking.

"Keep trying," she coaxes me

I try with all my might, thinking once again that nothing is happening, but she says, "There! It moved a little."

"Really, I still don't feel anything."

"It may take a little longer. I checked with the anesthesiologist, and he said sometimes it can take up to two hours for feeling to return."

I am slightly relieved. At least I know my toe is starting to work again. The nurses start to discuss moving me up to my room. There are more surgeries taking place, and they need the recovery area cleared out for new patients. "When can I see my baby?" I ask again. I have to see him. I have to have some sense that a baby really was born. It all feels so surreal. They discuss wheeling my bed down to the NICU for a minute on the way to my room but decide against it. The morning is busy, and they all have much to do. I want to scream, "I don't care how busy you are! Just let me see my baby!"

We reach my room on the third floor, and Shawn and I are left alone for a moment. Our eyes are wide with fear and uncertainty. A motherly nurse with a kind face enters and introduces herself, giving us information and instruction, but I don't really hear her.

I begin crying and ask, "When can I see my baby?"

She looks at me with compassion and says, "Well, you're supposed to be on bed rest for a full twelve hours post surgery, but after you regain full feeling in your legs, I'll get you in a wheelchair and take you down to the NICU. You'll only be able to stay for ten or fifteeen minutes, though, and then we have to get you back into bed. I'll take you down one more time later this afternoon as well."

I'm so thankful for her. Finally, someone is giving me an answer. I pray the spinal wears off quickly. The nurse leaves us alone, and the weight of what has just happened begins to press down on us.

Shawn and I look at each other, and the tears begin to flow freely. Our entire world has been turned upside down.

Soon Major Cheryl arrives from The Salvation Army. She walks into the room, eyes full of concern. I look at her and try to speak, but all that comes out is wracking sobs. My body is still shaking. I still feel numb in my legs. I've never felt so completely out of control in my entire life. She begins crying as well, telling us she loves us and everything is going to be okay. I appreciate her presence and her tears of compassion, but her words feel so hollow. How can everything possibly be okay?...

Part Two:

Grandma Jan's Journal

A Special Poem

February 24, 2009

Budding baby boy
Enveloped in Spirit
New in hope and brimming with
Joy
Anew each day:
Mindful and merry,
Insight of the ages, a
New man for the times. He will

Lead and
Enrich lives with his
Effervescent personality

How I Love Him Already! (May 2009)

Author's note: During Benjamin's NICU stay, I was so physically and emotionally exhausted that keeping a written record of events was one of the furthest things from my mind. Thankfully, my mom, Janis, kept a written account during that time via e-mails to family and friends and through her own personal journal entries. A few months later she sent me a typed copy of it all, lovingly entitled "Grandma Jan's Journal." I am dedicating this section of the book to include excerpts from her writings, in order to fill in gaps and details that I would have surely missed otherwise. I'm sure you will enjoy her honesty, wisdom, and occasional humor as she tells this portion of our story through the eyes of a loving mother and grandmother. Thanks, Mom!

******

May, 22 2009

Benjamin was born at 5:39 a.m. by C-section. He weighs 7 lb 6.4 oz and is 19 inches long. He is on a ventilator to help him breathe, and his blood pressure is low. An ultrasound of his heart and genetic testing have already been done, results to be in on Tuesday.

Dana is heartbroken over not getting to hold him yet. It helped her to see him, touch him, and talk to him. She is still queasy from the surgery but stopped shaking after two hours. Shawn is a calm, stable presence.

My writing here sounds wooden, perhaps reflecting my numbed emotions. I am afraid.

Last night, though, about 9:30 p.m., God spoke to me through a verse from my daily reading that reminded me, again, that He is in charge of the details and that we can trust Him. That sudden awareness brought a surge of joy as I prayed for a surge of energy for Dana.

Oh, and another important detail. The cord was looped around Benjamin's neck, so it is a good thing they did the C-section.

What am I hoping? That the breathing issue resolves quickly and turns out to be a typical breathing issue for C-section births. That his blood pressure improves. That his enlarged heart is not serious. That the genetic testing comes out normal. That even if these hopes are not granted that Dana and Shawn will not lose faith or become bitter. My hope (you can read prayer interchangeably for that word) is for Benjamin to have a full, loving, productive life, fulfilling God's plans for him.

It is hard to see my child going through the most difficult part of parenthood already—wanting desperately to make things better for her baby, wanting to hold him and nurse him, wanting to simply be with him, feeling out of control. God, help her and Shawn. Help me to have a steadying, calm presence for them, unhindered, confident, listening, loving. This is hard. Please use me to be a blessing to them and to Benjamin…

******

May 23, 2009 (11 a.m. visit with Benjamin)

What a sweet, tender picture of faith, Dana and Shawn talking to Benjamin as they touch him. Dana read some verses from Psalms and Proverbs and sang a little.

******

May 23 (evening)

Looking at Benjamin from the side Shawn usually stands at (Benjamin's head to my left), I see it all at once. I say nothing as the evidence seems to grow before my eyes: the deeply creased palm line, the almost nonexistent neck, the almond eyes, the rounded face, the ears up tight and somehow a little different against his head.

To me, the prophetic words said over him make sense in a new configuration. He will be a shining light, a person of faith, an inspiration because of the totality of who he is, which includes Down syndrome.

******

May 24, 2009

I was so sure that a cesarean was the wrong thing for Dana. Feeling a surge of the Spirit, I prayed for a surge of energy for her. But she ended up with a cesarean eight hours later, a decision that probably saved Benjamin's life because the cord was wrapped around his neck.

I may have the best intentions, but I get it wrong so often. What feels so sure in my heart can turn out to be plain old wrong. What I worried about was whether or not she had the baby vaginally; I thought that was the issue at hand, and I thought I had the answer. But God knew differently.

It was His Spirit that gave me peace; it was His Spirit that led me to pray for an energy surge for Dana. However, my interpretation of what that meant turned out to be different than His intent. I thought I was praying for a natural birth, but perhaps what God was leading me to pray for was something entirely different.

Now that Benjamin is here and facing so many challenges, Dana needs a surge of the Spirit and a surge of energy for this time of uncertainty and waiting. She and Shawn will need still more if Benjamin has special needs.

All I know to pray for now is God's will, God's grace. But God will be faithful. I just don't know what that will look like yet.

******

May 26, 2009

Benjamin's oxygen level has been in the 30's today. He was taken off the bilirubin lights and his color looks much better. He is absolutely the sweetest little guy. I marvel over every little twitch or grimace he makes.

I love him for exactly who he is. Whatever challenges he faces with Down syndrome make no difference; Benjamin is who God made him to be, and many blessings will come through him.

Tomorrow we find out about the echocardiogram results…God, please protect and keep our little Benjamin safe. Bring the healing that You will. Give us strength for each day and each moment.

******

May 27, 2009 (Dana's 27th birthday)

Here is the (doctor's report) summary:

Benjamin has a ventricular septal defect (VSD) in his heart that will likely require surgery eventually. The problem with the aorta (?) seems to have been resolved by the medication. A possible problem from that medication is renal failure, which started up with him, so she (doctor) stopped that medication. His kidneys are starting to function again. He is peeing well.

The bloated belly is at least partly related to the kidney problem but should resolve itself. The kidney problem is called mild hydronephrosis.

With the heart problems, Benjamin has a mild pericardial effusion.

The doctor is going to try to encourage him to breathe more on his own with caffeine. Right now the respirator is doing most of the work, a typical scenario for a preemie. The morphine he's been getting also contributes to depending on the respirator.

He was also given steroids over the weekend, which have helped. (I don't remember with what). The heart problem is typical for Down syndrome.

The doctor is going to start giving Benjamin Dana's colostrum through the tubing today, about a teaspoon. That will be gradually increased as he tolerates it.

Before Dana can hold him, he must be off the respirator and have the lines through his belly button removed. Those will be replaced by a pick line inserted in his arms or leg for IVs.

He has made progress, and though he is still sick, he is not as sick as he was a couple of days ago. He will need to be followed by a cardiologist for his whole life.

To me the report was encouraging because it showed he has made improvement, and the doctor explained that problems and process in detail so we could understand.

Dana's milk has come in. I am concerned about her getting too engorged. The doctor's report was hard for her, hard for Shawn, too, but I can't read his emotions like I can hers.

Before we came in this morning, I was pleased that Dana decided we can go home with Shawn tomorrow when he has to go in to work. She wants to pick up more clothing. She is accepting the idea that we may be here for a few weeks rather than a few days.

May 29, 2009

Benjamin continues to make progress. He was taken off the ventilator yesterday and is now on the CPAP machine, which means he is doing the work of breathing all on his own with the oxygen supplement. His tummy continues to get smaller, though the doctor says he will simply have a big belly! They will attempt again today to put a pick line in—then the tubes into his belly button will be able to be removed and Dana and Shawn can hold him. This morning we saw him get ¾ ounce of Dana's milk through his tube. Results of the echocardiogram that was done this morning will be in today or tomorrow. The doctor says he looks good and is improving…His color is good. How I love him already.

******

May 29 e-mail: The First Week

Dear Friends,

We have so much to be grateful for. I'd like to recap highlights of the past week for you.

Because fetal monitoring showed Benjamin to be in some distress, Dana's labor was induced last Thursday in her 35th week of pregnancy. The decision for a C-section was made early Friday morning. Benjamin Lee Hemminger arrived at 5:39 a.m. on May 22, weighing in at 7.64 pounds and 19 inches long. (Yes, he's a chunk!) Immediately after birth he showed signs of respiratory distress and was whisked off to NICU.

Shawn got to see him get cleaned up and take a few initial pictures. Dana waited four very long hours before she got to see him. (It was supposed to be twelve hours, but the nurses bent the rules for her.)

I saw Benjamin for the first time less than 24 hours after he was born. By then, of course, he was hooked up to multiple monitors, tubes, and the ventilator. God's grace was there for me because none of that bothered me. I was (and am) simply so grateful to see my beautiful new grandson and be here for Dana and Shawn. It was an added blessing when Shawn's mother, Cyndi, arrived the next day. Cyndi and I make a very good grandma team!

There were a few rough days in which everything seemed to go wrong for Benjamin. His oxygen had to be increased, his belly began to bloat, and he had to be catheterized. The medicine given him for his heart caused his kidneys to start to shut down. He had to have an echocardiogram to diagnose his heart problems (which may require surgery in a couple years), and for a brief time it was thought he might need abdominal surgery.

Things started to turn around by Monday, and he has made major improvement since then. He is our little fighter! Yesterday he was taken off the ventilator and is now on a CPAP machine. His bloating is subsiding, and he peed the catheter out yesterday. He is being fed Dana's breast milk through his gastric tube—3/4 ounce this morning!

After several unsuccessful attempts yesterday by other nurses, today's nurse, "the queen of pick lines" managed to get one in by his foot (his chubby little arms didn't cooperate) which will mean that Dana and Shawn will finally get to hold him, I hope tomorrow. After he is introduced to a bottle, Dana can start breastfeeding him. In the meantime, she is faithfully pumping every three hours. The lactation specialists are very knowledgeable and helpful.

Benjamin is more precious than I can say. With the ventilator out, he can finally cry. I got to hear him when Shawn changed his diaper today. I can say with full assurance that Dana and Shawn will be (and are already) extra special parents for their extra *special baby. Benjamin has Down syndrome, confirmed by genetic testing last week. We love him so much, right down to his 47th chromosome.*

Please keep Benjamin, Shawn, and Dana in your prayers. There will be challenges ahead, I am sure, but I am also sure of God's tender love for all of us. I know that I am totally smitten with my grandson.

Love,

Grandma Jan

******

May, 30 2009

Dana got to hold Benjamin today! He is off the CPAP and on oxygen through his nose. The nurse on duty is the one who was their nurse in labor.

Shawn is very wise, suggesting we set up a basic schedule for each day to help us eat at regular times and make sure Dana gets a daily nap. Her milk production was down yesterday from doing too much the day before. Last night I paid to rent a hospital breast pump so she can pump both sides at once.

This afternoon when Dana and Shawn went to see Benjamin, the nurse had him on his tummy for a while. He surprised them by lifting his head straight up, an amazing feat for a newborn anyway, but extra spectacular for a preemie with Down syndrome. He's a strong little boy, so determined, a real fighter.

Grandma's Ramblings (June 2009)

June 1, 2009

It's been a busy day.

Benjamin took his first bottle feeding. The physical therapist says he has a good, strong sucking reflex, but he's not sure what to do with the milk once it's in his mouth! Dana did her first skin-to-skin contact last night, and Benjamin wasn't sure what to do about that, either. He kept burying his nose in her chest (she was holding him upright as instructed) and lifting his head up. The physical therapist suggested her letting him suckle at her breast when it's empty, holding him swaddled since he flails around so much. I'm anxiously waiting to see him—it's 4:30 p.m. and I haven't had the chance to see him since yesterday morning.

Last night we drove to Dewey, picked up the second car, and spent the night at the house. Shawn left early this morning for work. It's the first week of summer day camp, and he's the director, so he really has to work this week. Dana and I took the big car back to Tulsa—I'm proud of myself for driving that boat! I dropped her off at the hospital and went to get us checked out of the Ronald McDonald house. Lots of trips to the car; I'm glad we moved most of the stuff last night. The anticipated opening at The Hospitality House came through, and we've checked in there…

What a ministry there is in providing shelter for families with a medical crisis. The Hospitality House is only a couple blocks from Hillcrest Hospital, which will help a lot. It is a faith-based non-profit…We are met with graciousness at every turn. God is taking such good care of us through these ministries and people, church friends, and hospital staff.

June 2 e-mail

Dana and I are settled in at The Hospitality House, a Christian ministry across the street from Hillcrest Hospital. THH has seven apartments, and dinners are provided every night. It's so nice to be closer to the hospital. Shawn will be coming down for the night after work today.

The speech therapist and the physical therapist came to give Benjamin a bottle feeding today. The PT said he did better than yesterday—he's getting the hang of sucking (which he does very well) and swallowing and breathing (getting those coordinated a bit better). Tomorrow the lactation consultant will come to help Dana with non-nutritive feeding—doing the initial breastfeeding session after she has pumped. This is to introduce Benjamin to latching on.

The doctor will have Benjamin's pick line taken out today since he's digesting the breast milk so well. Each little step brings us closer to the time we will get to bring him home.

We delight in every little grimace, sound, and squirm he makes. He is such a beautiful boy.

******

June 3, 2009

Dana's expectations were dashed this morning when Benjamin pretty much slept through the first latching on lesson. Naturally, she had hoped for an instantaneous response, but that is not what happened. Over lunch, she cried a bit, and I listened. I'm so grateful to have recently done the listening class in the Stephen Ministries training; that reminded me to keep my ears opened and my mouth closed.

Expectations are a funny thing. They seem so simple and straightforward, like clear indicators of the future. But so often what we picture in our minds doesn't even closely resemble reality. Without realizing it, we interpret God's promises into our own limited framework. Yes, we should live in expectation as well as the fullness of the present. We just need to remember that what we imagine is not always exactly what God has in mind.

Standing in the doorway, I start to cough. "Dana," I gasp, choking, "I need to learn not to swallow and breathe at the same time."

"Maybe that's where Benjamin gets it from."

So already I have something vital in common with my grandson: we both need to learn how to coordinate breathing and swallowing. Let's hope he learns more quickly than I have.

"Dana, guess what? I won a spitting contest!"

Those were Shawn's first words when Dana called him tonight. An image rises in my mind of Benjamin as a laughing little boy coached by his daddy in the fine art of spitting watermelon seeds.

What a blessed boy Benjamin is. With Mommy and Daddy's loving care and spiritual nurture, he will be himself, exactly as God intends him to be. I see laughter and love, giggles and smiles, generosity and grace, sincere faith and full trust in Jesus.

And who knows? He may even become the family champion of spitting contests.

******

June 4 e-mail: Grandma's Big Moment

I got to hold Benjamin for the first time today—thirty minutes of bliss.

The lactation consultant came in to work with mama and baby again today while Benjamin was awake and alert. He successfully latched on several times and looked rather surprised when he got some milk. Dana has the "okay" from the doctor to do a session a day whenever Benjamin is awake. The lactation consultant was very pleased with Benjamin's response.

A pleasant surprise when we came in this morning was that Benjamin has been moved out of a heat warmer bed and into a regular baby bed on wheels.

I'm going to be smiling all day as I think about holding my sweet grandson and seeing him start learning to nurse.

Each day brings another little milestone along the way toward bringing him home…

******

June 5 e-mail: Rumbles and Rambles

Dana had her two week check-up today and is doing very well. Benjamin has been moved up to three bottle feedings a day from one (the others are through his gastric tube). Dana will do her daily nursing "practice" with him this evening. Shawn will be here for the weekend.

I love watching Benjamin wake up. He starts with raised eyebrows, then moves to opening one eye, then the other. These steps are repeated with little nap breaks in between. Finally, both eyes open, and they are such a deep blue. He looks all around, very alert and attentive.

Like his daddy, he never sneezes just once. The magic number seems to be five.

He definitely does not appreciate diaper changes and surprised his mommy yesterday with a rumble and a spray as she changed his diaper. He usually hollers his head off and has his arms and legs in perpetual motion.

That's probably enough of Grandma's ramblings for now. We're going back to the apartment soon for our daily nap.

******

June 10 e-mail:

The big news today is that Benjamin's feeding schedule is up to four bottle or breastfeeding sessions and four tube feedings each day. That meant that Dana got to nurse him twice today. He's an old pro now.

Benjamin is a boy of many talents, and one of them is requiring about three diapers per changing. I am on my best grandma behavior and have not changed a single diaper yet. I serve as the cheerleader. ("Go, Benjamin, go!")

Please continue your prayers that he will be able to come home soon. We're eagerly anticipating sleepless nights, mounds of diapers, and loads of laundry. And then maybe I'll get to hold him more often, too, though I intend to graciously hand him over whenever it's diaper time.

June 11 e-mail: Eating My Words

Benjamin wouldn't wake up to nurse so I suggested changing his diaper again, which makes him really mad. (He had a rumble right after the last diaper change minutes ago.)

Let's just say that I was doubly impressed by Dana's diaper changing skills when I changed him. He has the wiggle, squirm and kick routine down very well. Add to that the various wires and monitors that like to get tangled down around his feet, and the uncooperative snaps to his sleeper. But I managed, and he woke up mad, so my mission was accomplished.

******

June 12 e-mail: Ah, Benjamin

This morning, the doctor wrote the orders for Benjamin's feeding schedule to go from six to eight. That means no more feeding tube. It could also mean that he will be able to come home early next week…

Benjamin is three weeks old today. He is still on oxygen, and we are praying that he will be able to come off that entirely and soon. (He can be sent home on it, though.) His heart is working well despite the holes…The doctor thinks that his lungs have a little inflammation left over, which is causing the need for the oxygen.

I have a perpetual smile on my face, thinking about my sweet grandson and thanking God for all He has done and is doing for this lovely little boy.

June 14, 2009

Eight bottles and counting…Even though Benjamin's oxygen remains right around thirty percent, he may be coming home this week. I believe all he has to do is pass the car seat test.

Having my grandson in the NICU these first weeks of his life has taught me many things I never expected to learn. I prefer learning in a structured environment, but this has been learning on the go. Some of the learning has come from doctors and nurses, some from other parents and grandparents, some from reading. There is only one thing I did not have to learn from an outside source: loving Benjamin.

To see him is to love him. I know his lengthy wake-up ritual that spreads out over twenty minutes or more: raising his eyebrows as if in a mighty effort to get those eyelids unstuck; scrunching up his face as if to cry; squirming around within his swaddled blankets. And then after a few more eyebrow raises and torso wiggles his eyes pop open: deep blue, bright, alert almond eyes looking all around; eyes that communicate interest; gazing and darting eyes that remind me of a little bird; those eyes that showed confusion and surprise the first time Dana introduced him to her breast.

The last time in my life that I was so smitten with love was for my own babies. Now I watch Dana taking in every little movement and grimace, delighting in every smile or frown, giggling with the sprays and rumbles that accompany most diaper changes. It is deeply satisfying to watch my child comforting and nurturing her child.

I hope, of course, that Benjamin will pass his car seat test the first time: he must maintain good vital signs sitting in the car seat for an hour—the duration of our drive home to Dewey. I hope even more that he will learn to prefer breast to bottle, and that he can suckle well enough to not need the formula supplementation the doctor wants him to have. I envision love and laughter as this little guy grows at his unique pace and develops his unique personality.

Adorable is the word for Benjamin. He makes this grandma smile every day.

******

June 15 e-mail: Soon

Benjamin will be coming home on Wednesday!

We are hoping he will be able to come off the last little bit of oxygen tomorrow. They tried taking him off today but the timing was lousy—just before his circumcision. He has nursed very well today, though, and he will be able to come home even if he has to be on oxygen.

He is awake and alert so much more now. When he is hollering his head off over a diaper change, we remind him that it won't take so long at home without wires and without having to take his blood pressure and temperature every time. Once his diaper is changed, though, he quiets right down and looks all around with those sweet blue eyes.

We appreciate your continuing prayers as we make the adjustment from hospital to home…and as I make the adjustment of leaving in a week and a half or so.

******

June 17, 2009

Benjamin came home today!

June 19, 2009

"Pick up his feet! Pick up his feet!"

Shawn's advice is good, but Dana is a second too late. Benjamin has just begun his first bath at home by pooping and sticking his feet in it.

The preparations for the bath take much longer than the bath itself. The brand-new baby towels and washcloths must be washed and dried by Grandma before first use. Mommy and Daddy carefully plot out their plan: a sponge bath with baby lying in the ducky mesh of the baby tub.

Just a couple minutes after the poo, bath time is done. Instead of crying, Benjamin just looks around, probably content to have already left his mark on this milestone. Once he is dressed in his brand new outfit, though, maybe he will leave another mark. But at least this time his diaper will be on.

******

June 21, 2009

"You fight me and then you complain that you're not getting any milk!"

Those words from Dana to Benjamin make me wonder how often God says the same to us with the same loving, exasperated tone.

Sometimes Benjamin fights the breast. He is desperately hungry but pushes away from Mommy even as he tries to nurse. He arches his head back, pushes with his arm, and cries as he removes himself from his source of nourishment. Fortunately, his mother is both gentle and persistent, knowing he needs her even when he resists.

As God's offspring, how often do we push our source of spiritual nourishment away? We fight against our Father's nurture even as we angrily demand it. Fortunately, God is both gentle and persistent, knowing our need of Him even though we resist His care.

******

June 24 e-mail: Update

Benjamin survives this heat wave better than I do! He's on the tiniest bit of oxygen; we're hoping his Friday appointment with the pediatrician will result in no more oxygen tanks and tubes.

He is thriving: nursing, sleeping, and eliminating well…There are a number of stories on that last one already! In the next few weeks he has appointments with a pediatric ophthalmologist and a cardiologist. He is a very easy baby—I can't get used to the concept of waking him up for feedings, though he usually wakes up on his own, and him being happy whether he is held or put down. If he is not hungry, he doesn't mind diaper changes, though he is a regular little wiggle worm, looking around, bicycling with his feet, waving his arms.

Dana and Shawn have received many wonderful blessings from friends and work and church. While we were in Tulsa, people took care of their dogs, mowed their lawn, and cleaned the house. We were taken out to eat multiple times, checks and cash were lovingly given, and The Salvation Army has rallied volunteers to provide evening meals since we got home.

The application for early intervention services for Benjamin (called Sooner Start) will get underway next week…

Shawn's family gets here for a one week visit this Friday. I'll be flying to Denver on June 29 and driving down to Colorado Springs to visit my son. My flight back to Seattle is on July 4.

Thank you so much for all of your kind thoughts and prayers.

Best Picture

July 1 e-mail: Best Picture

Dear Friends,

I'm sitting in the Tully's Coffee shop in King Sooper's on Academy Boulevard in Colorado Springs. And, of course, I'm thinking about Benjamin. The attached picture shows him on the changing table, finally off oxygen. Isn't he a cutie? However, I feel none of the pictures I have do him justice. To get the real sense of Benjamin, you have to hold him, see his wake-up routine, watch his expressions, look into his blue eyes, and listen for the telltale rumbles that will tell you it is time to visit the changing table again.

As of last Friday, he is off oxygen. He weighed in at 8 lb 15 oz, so he is thriving. The pediatrician could not detect a heart murmur. Dana and Shawn will be taking Benjamin to Tulsa to see the cardiologist on July 6 to get his heart officially checked again. I will keep you appraised of his progress.

I've learned something about myself. In the past, when I would see a person with Down syndrome, that is all I would see. Now, when I look at my grandson, I see a unique and much-loved person. The stereotyping is gone. I could not be prouder of my grandson.

Whenever Benjamin comes to mind, say a prayer for him and his parents. Dana and Shawn are blessed to have him, and he is blessed to have them.

A Note from Grandma Jan

Love at First Sight

It was love at first sight and, boy, was he a sight. Seven and a half pounds of sweetness lay there in the heated crib, tubes and wires snaking out from him, the ventilator like a stake down his throat. Sedated, he slept, unresponsive to our tentative touches.

Actually, it was love before first sight, love born in the joyful weeping of my daughter's announcement: "I'm pregnant." I loved Benjamin before I knew he was Benjamin. I loved him when I visited my daughter, proud with her cute five-month tummy. I loved him when I saw her blooming belly profiles at seven and eight months. I loved him when the scary news came about induced premature labor and caesarean section. I loved him, wishing the holes could be in my heart, not his. And I loved him as I saw the signs of Down syndrome in his sweet almond eyes and unbroken lifelines across his wide palms.

I held him for the first time when he was about four weeks old as Dana left his NICU bedside for the mommy room to pump milk. (The nurse bent the rules for me.) I held him at Shawn and Dana's home, the oxygen cord snaking across the room, the heart monitor letting out its scary blips and bleeps. I held him after my sister died in October 2009, savoring his sweet baby weight that soothed and healed.

Benjamin doesn't have to do anything to earn my love. I love him because he is. I love him without knowing exactly who he will be. I delight in his unfolding personality. I'll love him through good times and bad. He will never have to doubt that I love him. Every time I see him, I fall in love with him all over again and ponder the enormity of God's grace and the infinity of His love for each of us.

Part Three:

Stories & Reflections from a Mother's Heart

Broken

As a young college student, I walked through a season of heartbreak that drove me to draw nearer to Jesus. I wrote quite a bit of poetry during that time as an outlet for the many emotions swirling inside of me. The poems often started out in sorrow but ended in worship and prayer. I was amazed at how the Lord met me each time as the words seemed to take on a life of their own. Years later, in the midst of more swirling emotions concerning my son, I picked up one of my poems and was overwhelmed that the words flowing out of me as a 20 year old, in a completely different set of circumstances, could still minister so deeply to my heart in my present state. The following poem, with only minor revisions from its original draft, is my life-long prayer:

My defeated, grieving heart, eyes stained red with tears

Yet on Your altar of grace I have chosen to lay down my fears.

My dreams I had clutched so tightly; the heart is so deceiving.

Thinking I knew the way to walk I kept myself believing

That the truth I had perceived must be the only way

When the true desire of Your heart is for me to humbly pray.

What I had seen as beauty, You knew could soon be shaken.

In love You'll never rest until I am completely taken

Into the deepness of Your heart where my identity is placed

In the promise of Your Cross and the fullness of Your grace.

My broken pieces belong to You; do with them as You will.

And as You overtake me in Your peace may I be still.

This life is Yours, not mine. You are the Lord of all.

Direct my path with every step, and catch me when I fall.

Burn away my self 'til all is stripped away.
May I live in brokenness each and every day.
For there true beauty resides; Your richness fills my soul.
As I step into Your Presence, I know I am made whole.
Oh, my precious Jesus, Your face is all I seek.
I rejoice that You are strong every place that I am weak.

I love to stand before You. I want to live before Your eyes.
Guard me from the enemy; free me from all of his lies.
One day I will be with You; I'll gaze into Your face.
I ache to feel the fullness of that tender, intimate embrace.
But until that Day arrives, You are my daily food.
Please take my broken pieces and feed a multitude
So that I may stand before You, knowing I did not live in vain.
You are a Sovereign God, and I surrender to You my pain
That You may form beauty from ashes and build within me a fire
Spreading out to those around me as I burn with Your desire.

May the "broken pieces" of these following pages offer nourishment to your soul…

First Glimpse

My first glimpse of him was so surreal. After the numbness of the spinal finally wore off, and I'd had some more time to rest, our kind nurse helped me into a wheelchair and took Shawn and me down to the NICU. The pain at my C-section incision site was very real, but the pain in my heart was greater. I could take medicine to help soothe the pain in my abdomen, but my heart was torn and bleeding with no apparent remedy. I tried to take in all the surroundings. We had our own little corner of the NICU with a curtain that could be drawn for privacy. Intimidating medical equipment and monitors were all around, the constant beeping putting my nerves even more on edge. I was grateful, though, for the individual sign that had already been made for Benjamin and taped to the front of his small bed. His name was attached with white foam letters on a blue background, decorated with a foam basketball and soccer ball, and stamped with his tiny footprints right in the center. It gave a small sense of warmth to an otherwise sterile environment.

Was this really my baby? His still, ashy body was hooked up to so many tubes and wires-the only sign of life was the gentle rising and falling of his chest, but the ventilator was doing most of the work for him. I gingerly reached out and touched his little hand. I don't remember what I said to him, but I know I tried to speak peace and love amid all the shock and fear swirling inside of me. At one point (either that visit or a later one) I asked the nurse if it would be okay to kiss Benjamin's hand. She seemed surprised and told me, "Of course." Though it hurt to bend down, I touched his tiny hand to my lips, longing for some sort of connection with my son. It felt as though the visit was over as soon as it started, and it was time to be wheeled back up to the hospital room.

In the days following, the scene was much the same, though as my body began to recover, I walked more and rode in the wheelchair less. My arms ached to hold my son, but I was given no definite time frame of when I could. He had to be weaned off the ventilator, which felt like such a slow process--two steps forward, one step back. He had to have the delicate IVs attached directly into his belly button removed and a pick line inserted. This was no easy task. The many failed attempts were evident as little red dots all over his arms and legs. My only consolation was that in his sedated state, Benjamin probably didn't feel the pokes. I knew he was my baby, but he didn't feel like my baby. A bond had not yet been formed. I missed the feeling of him inside my womb. I felt connected then; I felt like he knew who I was then. I hoped he could recognize my voice and know that Mommy was near.

The anticipated day finally arrived, May 30, 2009. It had been nine days since Benjamin's delivery, but it felt like a short life-time already. I had already been discharged from the hospital and was staying with my mom at the Ronald McDonald house about fifteen minutes away. My mother-in-law Cyndi had been with us for a few days but had to return to Minnesota. Shawn already had to return home for work and was making the hour-long drive to see us as much as he could. Later, Mom and I would move to the Hospitality House only two blocks away from the hospital. My 27th birthday had been a few days before. It was the hardest birthday of my life. All I wanted was to hold my son, but my request could not yet be granted. Benjamin's gift to me that day, however, was to open his eyes so I could see them for the first time. Now the moment had finally arrived. I sat in the rocking chair eagerly waiting as the nurse swaddled Benjamin and tried not to tangle his tubes and wires too much. My first experience of having him in my arms was beautiful. This really was my baby! Shortly thereafter we tried our first attempt at "kangaroo care," the important skin-to-skin contact that a newborn baby needs. The first session was disappointing.

Benjamin was in an unfamiliar position and spent most of the time wiggling around, trying to make sense of everything. The second time was sweet, as he relaxed into my body and we rocked.

I could never hold him long enough. All too soon it would be time to put him back in his NICU crib and say our goodbyes. Every parting was painful, even if it was only for a few hours. I would kiss and kiss and kiss his face, wanting to savor every moment with my son. Shawn and I would read scripture over him, pray over him, and I would sing over him. There was so little we could do for his physical care at that point, but we could make sure Benjamin knew he was loved. The thought of being able to hold him without tubes and wires away from the sterile environment of the NICU seemed glorious and almost too good to be true. This was the only world my son knew at this point, and I so wanted him to see the beauty of the outdoors, the comfort of our home and especially his nursery, lovingly prepared just for him…

Now fast forward several months. Benjamin did get to come home on June 17, 2009, 27 days after he was born. Though there were more hospital stays in time, life really did fall into a rhythm as we settled into our new life with our son. All during my pregnancy we prayed for a cuddly baby. God answered our prayer! At the time I write this Benjamin is fast approaching his second birthday, and he is a Momma's boy! When I hold him facing me, his face lights up in a huge smile, and he often lets out a squeal. We make faces back and forth to each other. One of his favorite games is for me to kiss him all over his neck while he holds his head back and erupts into delighted giggles. In a desire to return my kisses, he will lick me across the face. He is such a cuddly guy that it is often difficult to get things done. He holds out his arms to me and fusses until I pick him up. Sometimes in exasperation I find myself saying "Mommy doesn't have to hold you *all* the time!" I am often caught by the irony of my own words. I remember the days where I longed to hold my son and wasn't able to or the days when I would hold him in the NICU rocker but it was never long enough. Even as I've tried to write my thoughts today, we've had to take some "cuddle breaks," and I can hear the discontentment beginning to rise again. In these moments I must remind myself what a privilege it is to hold Benjamin in my arms, what a privilege it is to have him safe at home with me, what a privilege it is to be his mommy.

Projectile Poop!

It had been a really emotional day. Shawn was visiting us in Tulsa for the weekend and would have to return home in the morning. We were still unsure of how long Benjamin would be in the NICU, and the stress of not being able to be together as a family was taking its toll. There had been many tears that day, and we were dreading the morning when we would have to say goodbye again. For Shawn it was especially difficult, as he had to be separated from me and Benjamin.

While spending time in the NICU that evening, Shawn took his turn at diaper duty. Now, for anyone who has ever had to change a diaper for a baby in the NICU, you know that it takes some extra skill and patience, especially if you're not used to changing diapers to begin with! First, you have a limited space to work in. The NICU crib was basically a small plastic tub with padding on the bottom. Next, take into account the multiple tubes and wires, some of which are attached to the baby's feet. If you couple those things with the natural wiggles of a newborn, you have a potential recipe for a big mess!

On this particular evening, Shawn forgot the nurse's advice to change the diaper from the *side* of the crib and decided to stand at the *foot* of the crib, placing himself directly in the line of fire. He was already frazzled from the emotional stress of the day, the complications of the diaper change, and the cries of a discontented baby, when Benjamin decided it was time to unleash a powerful bowel movement. When I say powerful, I mean it had air time! The yellow and watery stool of a breastfed infant exploded from our small son, spraying the foot of the crib, splattering all over Daddy's shirt and even hitting Mommy's bag on the floor! In complete shock and disgust, Shawn leaped back with a cry. For him, this was the last straw for his already raw nerves. With no attempt to conceal his irritation, he announced that he was going to change and would return shortly. As I took over diaper duty, my tears flowed freely, though these were tears brought on by uncontrollable laughter—wonderfully refreshing after the previous tears of the day.

I don't remember much of what happened during the rest of that evening. Shawn returned with fresh clothes, feeling a little bit calmer. I probably continued to giggle throughout the evening, each time I remembered the expression on Shawn's face at the moment of impact! I think Benjamin knew Mommy needed to laugh that day. (Shawn can laugh about the incident now too). I do know that Benjamin has never again graced us with the impressive "projectile poop" as we have come to call it. However, his favorite opportunity to release a bowel movement continues to be in the *middle* of a diaper change!

"Sighting Day"

During Benjamin's first month at home I was in a fog, trying to get into a rhythm with our brand new life and my brand new schedule. Our little baby slept most of the time, largely due to the three holes in his heart that had yet to be repaired. I would often have to wake him up just to get him to eat. I wanted interaction with my son in addition to our nursing times, so every day for the first few weeks I would lay him on a Boppy pillow on my lap and read to him. He would often fall back asleep or quietly look around, but I cherished the time.

During Shawn's and my dating years, we were introduced to an amazing children's book trilogy (*Tales of the Kingdom; Tales of the Resistance; Tales of the Restoration*) by David and Karen Mains. Each book contains a collection of stories that are rich with allegory about the Kingdom of God, expressing His heart with creativity and excellence. In the first book *Tales of the Kingdom* the subjects of the King (Jesus) live in Great Park, tended by Caretaker (Holy Spirit) and His wife Mercie. On a regular basis, the people of Great Park come together for the Great Celebration—a night of feasting and festivity and fellowship with the King. In addition, the children regularly enjoy a day of fun and games called "Sighting Day." On this day, the King appears all around Great Park in many different disguises, and the children try to recognize Him in whatever form He presents Himself. Afterward, they spend the rest of the day playing together. It was while reading the story called "Sighting Day" to Benjamin in those early weeks, that I experienced an unexpected embrace from the Lord. While so much of that season is a fog in my mind, this particular memory stands out clearly.

As I neared the end of the story (which I had read many times before), I came to the part where Caretaker and a young boy visit

Outcast Village, a place reserved for those who had been wounded in the evil Enchanted City, and desperately needed Mercie's tender care. The following paragraph resonated in the core of my being, and the tears began to fall:

> *Caretaker explained that on Sighting Day many outcasts were unable to play the game of hunting the King. Some were wounded. Some were blinded. Others were mending from their diseases.* <u>*Instead the King came to them*</u>. *He sang songs and told stories. He wove moonlight and the warm night and all good things together until the hearts of the outcasts were comforted because the King had been among them* (underline mine).

It's hard to express the tender love and comfort that poured into my heart at that moment. I knew that I was one of the deeply wounded ones without the strength and energy to seek the King. Regardless of my present state, though, in His compassion King Jesus promised to *come to me*.

Since that day He's come to me in many ways, sometimes in the disguise of another person, an event, a song, a still, small voice…Sometimes He comes to me in a profound way that thrills and comforts my heart; often He comes in simple ways that I may not even always perceive. Many times He comes in ways I would not have expected or even chosen. Regardless of how He chooses to come, though, the point is that *He comes*. He is faithful. And the more Jesus comes to me in my brokenness, the more quickly I run to Him as I experience pain. He is my safe place.

> *And so the boy* [or girl!] *discovered that seek-the-King is a wonderful game. Like all games it must be played with a child's heart, which believes and is always prepared to be surprised, because a King can wear many disguises.*

Work Cited

Mains, David and Karen. *Tales of the Kingdom.* Waverly, PA: Lamplighter Publishing, 1983. 67-68.

A Mended Heart

It was one of the most difficult moments of my life. Shawn and I stood with our pastors, Majors Alan and Cheryl, in a hallway at St. Francis Children's Hospital in Tulsa, Oklahoma. In a few moments two-month-old Benjamin would be taken back for open heart surgery. I held him close to my chest, while two nurses patiently waited for us to give our son some final kisses and cuddles. With an aching heart, I handed my tiny baby to one of the nurses, not knowing when I would hold him again. She looked at me compassionately and assured me, "We'll take good care of him." I nodded in appreciation as the tears welled up in my eyes. After we watched the nurses disappear with Benjamin, we turned and walked the other direction to the waiting room where we would stay for the four-hour-long surgery. I felt like I was in a bad dream, but I knew I wasn't going to wake up. This was real.

It all started a week and a half prior on July 6, 2009. Benjamin had only been home for a little over two weeks when we took him to his first cardiologist appointment. After looking at our son's heart through an echocardiogram, Dr. Kimberling told us it was essential that Benjamin have surgery in the near future. If his condition was not treated within six months, it could become fatal. We were shocked and perplexed. Our son's pediatrician had not been able to detect the sound of a heart murmur. Dr. Kimberling explained that when the holes are very large, they often cannot be heard. What we had assumed was a positive sign was actually an indication of the severity of our baby's condition! He said he would discuss Benjamin's case with the heart surgeons at their meeting on Friday the tenth, and he would get back with us.

Shortly after that meeting, we received a call from Dr. Kimberling's office giving us a number to call to set up a consultation with the heart surgeons. I made the call on Monday the thirteenth, expecting to set up an appointment for discussion. Shawn was at work when I called, and my father-in-law D.J. was visiting but would be leaving in the morning to head back to MN. He was out getting a repair done on our car, so I was alone in the house with Benjamin. I was not prepared for the information I received on the other line. There was not time to set up a consultation. Dr. Nikaidoh, the best heart surgeon available, would be going out of town shortly, so the surgery needed to take place that week. In the numbness of my shock, I wrote down the necessary information. We needed to report to the hospital on Wednesday the fifteenth for pre-operation procedures and surgery would take place early the next morning. I was assured that this surgery was routine with a very low risk rate, and we could expect Benjamin to be discharged in five to eight days. I hung up the phone, the reality started to sink in, and the tears began to fall. I wasn't ready to have my son back in the hospital; he had only just come home. Through my tears I called Shawn and shared the news, which stunned him as well. Shortly after, D.J. returned to the house and presented me with a little Winnie the Pooh plush toy with a rattle inside that he'd picked up for his grandson. Fighting to contain my emotions, I told him what I had learned. He just listened, not knowing what to say. The next morning he was supposed to be on the road at 9:30 in the morning. Instead he held Benjamin for close to two hours, finally relinquishing him to me and heading out late in the morning.

The next day, before leaving for Tulsa, I sat nursing Benjamin in his nursery, knowing this would be one of the last times I would hold him to my breast before surgery. Benjamin was only clad in a diaper, so we could have some skin to skin contact. I looked down at his smooth little chest, knowing that the next time I sat here with my baby I would see a long scar. I had no idea how to process what we were about to walk through.

The afternoon was horrible. Benjamin had to have blood drawn for surgery, but due to his long stay in the NICU, all of his good veins had already been "tapped." It took four sets of people to finally get blood drawn from him. The first attempt was made by hospital nurses, the second attempt by pediatric nurses, the third attempt by a surgical assistant, and the fourth and finally successful attempt was by one of the heart surgeons herself--she had to make incisions in his hips. Due to the room's small space, we were finally asked to step outside, though we could come in to hold and comfort our son between the failed attempts. As we stood on the other side of the drawn curtain, Shawn and I held each other as the tears flowed, while we helplessly listened to our son's unbearable screams. We were completely drained, and we hadn't even gotten to surgery yet.

That night a good friend came into town and took us out for a nice dinner before we settled in to get a little bit of sleep at the Ronald McDonald house; I couldn't believe we were there again so soon. Before laying Benjamin down for the night, I nursed him one final time. He wasn't allowed anything after midnight, and I knew the morning would be difficult for him. As I lay down and tried to sleep, I felt the familiar beginnings of heartburn and acid reflux that had been plaguing me since shortly after Benjamin's birth. The first one hit me during Benjamin's first week home. It had been so scary and intense I went into a panic attack and had difficulty breathing, so Shawn drove me to the ER in the middle of the night while my mom stayed with our baby. As a nurse placed oxygen cannulas in my nose I said glumly, "My son wears these." I could read all of the monitors; they were depressingly familiar. I was treated for reflux and sent home. (It would be two more years before I would discover that I had been misdiagnosed. More on that later).

Back to the story: The late night meal and the overwhelming stress had triggered a major attack. I was up for the next several hours in misery, getting sick in the bathroom and feeling as though my chest and back were being repeatedly stabbed with blades. I cried and paced and prayed; this felt like too much to handle on the eve of my son's open heart surgery. When the symptoms finally began to subside, Benjamin began to stir. I held a pacifier to his mouth, hoping he would fall asleep again. When Shawn took over for me, I crawled into bed, hoping to get one or two hours of sleep before we had to take Benjamin to the hospital. I was exhausted.

After checking in at 5:00 am, we were directed to a room in the pre-surgery wing. It would be two hours before Benjamin was actually taken back for surgery. He was hungry and angry and screaming. In between trying to hold and comfort him and trying to listen to the nurses that came in and out, I somehow managed to doze off for a while. Soon, Majors Alan and Cheryl arrived to sit with us through our difficult day. We were so thankful for their presence. When it was finally near time for surgery, Dr. Nikaidoh came in to meet us, speak with us, and pray with us. An elderly Japanese man in excellent health, he is a world famous heart surgeon who has traveled the world teaching his own procedures. He is also a strong and incredibly humble Christian man, and he so encouraged and blessed our hearts as he prayed over our little boy, thanking God for His plans for Benjamin's life. We learned later that he will not begin anything in the surgery room until he and his team pray together. We were even more blessed to learn that Dr. Nikaidoh had only been in Tulsa for less than a year. We felt as though God had sent him for us, as I'm sure many families have felt since his arrival!

During the four hour wait, we were kept updated on Benjamin's progress through an hourly phone call sent directly to the waiting room. We were thankful for each good report. When surgery was completed, we were told we could stand in the hallway and watch them wheel our son by to the PICU, but we would have to remain in the waiting room a little bit longer before we could go join him. As we watched the surgical team pass by, we tried to get a glimpse of our baby, almost hidden in the giant hospital bed and array of tubes, wires, and bandages. When Dr. Nikaidoh saw us, he simply pointed to heaven and said, "He is good." Shortly after, he came to the waiting room with a hand-drawn diagram and explained Benjamin's surgery to us step by step. We could not have asked for a more excellent surgeon!

When we were finally able to join our son, we weren't quite prepared for what we would see. A large tube came out of his chest, draining excess blood from the surgery site. He was hooked up to countless tubes and wires—so many more than in the NICU. He was on a ventilator again and heavily sedated. We were told he would be on the ventilator for a day or two. However, due to complications with fluid retention and pulmonary hypertension, Benjamin remained on the ventilator for another nine days. His 5-8 day projected stay extended to a two week stay. It was a long two weeks. During the height of his fluid retention, we could hardly recognize our son; he was so puffy. My arms ached to hold him again, almost more intensely than they had the first week after his birth. I now knew what it felt like to hold him close to me, and I longed to hold him again. Though I wrestled with some guilt for not staying in the hospital with Benjamin, Shawn and I decided it would be best to stay in the Ronald McDonald house a block away, so I could get rest. I was exclusively pumping again, and I had to have rest to be able to maintain my supply of breast milk. The days were long and lonely since Shawn had to return to work, and he was not able to drive up to be with us every day, though he came as often as he could.

I filled the lengthy days with talking to my son, reading books, watching HGTV, pumping breast milk, and visiting with the PICU nurses and other families who had children in the PICU. The nurses and doctors were so loving and intentional with Benjamin. They clearly explained answers to all my questions and even offered information when I didn't ask any questions. One day I had some surprise visitors from a local support group called "Mended Little Hearts of Tulsa." They brought a gift bag and offered encouragement. Their visit was like a breath of fresh air. We also received so much love and support from family and friends, just as we had during Benjamin's NICU stay. We were surrounded with reminders of God's love.

Benjamin was finally well enough for his second home-coming on July 29, 2009. His chest scar healed beautifully, and he was such a bright-eyed and alert baby compared to his constant sleepy state before his surgery. The reports from his follow-up appointments with his cardiologist have been good. There is no reason to believe he will ever need another surgery. His heart has truly been mended!

A few months after we brought Benjamin home from surgery, some wonderful friends came over to talk with Shawn and me. They lovingly shared, "You have both been so wounded. You need to be intentional to seek healing for your hearts, so you don't get stuck in this place of grief." Their words resonated deep inside us both; we knew what they said was true. We simply existed day to day, numbed by our pain, confusion and disappointment. We had not lost our faith in God, but we weren't moving forward either. So, we took our friends' advice to heart and began to position ourselves before God, asking Him to heal us. We poured out to Him our emotions—anger, confusion, grief, fear, etc., knowing He was big enough to handle it all. We attended some weekend classes on healing the heart and mind that were offered at a church in

Tulsa. Most importantly, though, we set aside at least a few nights a week to just be still in the Lord's presence. We would pop in a worship CD, lay on the furniture or floor and just "soak." Often, it felt as though nothing was happening. Sometimes we would fall asleep. But, bit by bit, our hearts began to come alive again, and the thick fog began to clear.

Sometimes we would experience powerful things as we waited in the Lord's presence. The most significant incident for me happened one night as I lay on the couch and listened to the worship CD play. Suddenly the image of handing my baby to the nurse before surgery flooded my mind, and I felt the rawness of the pain again. In my heart I prayed, "Jesus, where were You in that moment?" In my mind's eye I suddenly saw myself handing Benjamin to Jesus, and He carried him back to surgery. My heart was overwhelmed, and as the tears flowed, I felt the sting of the memory begin to fade. The guilt I felt for not being with Benjamin 24/7 surfaced again as well, until I heard the Holy Spirit whisper to my heart, "I never left his bedside." Oh, how good my God is! He is full of compassion and so intimately aware of everything that concerns me. He loves my son so much more than I ever could, and the knowledge of His constant care for Benjamin has brought so much healing to my heart! In the natural, my son has a "mended little heart." In His patience and love, Jesus is in the process of mending mine. I know He is faithful to complete what He has started, and I am confident that He will never leave my side.

Another Hurdle

It was December 3, 2009, Shawn's 25th birthday. Unfortunately, I had a Christmas cantata practice that night, so after supper I headed to our church while Shawn stayed home with six-month-old Benjamin. I left a bottle of breast milk just in case and told him I would be back within a few hours. Practice went well, but I was anxious to be home with my husband on his birthday. As I pulled into the driveway and approached the front door, I heard the all too familiar screams of my son. I felt a mix of endearment for my baby who was probably anxious for the comfort of Mommy's breast and sympathy for Shawn, who hopefully hadn't been dealing with this the whole time. As I walked in the door I questioned, "How long has he been crying?"

"He just started a little while ago, but he won't take his bottle," was my husband's reply. I took Benjamin in my arms and headed for the rocking chair in the nursery, confident he would calm down as soon as he was able to nurse. To my surprise and concern, my baby would not even latch on to my breast, and continued to scream. That's when I noticed a look on his face I had not seen before. His eyes looked glassy and far-away, and his cry did not sound like a cry of hunger but a cry of pain. Alarmed, I called Shawn in to the room. We had no idea what was going on and were afraid that he may even be having a seizure. Shawn took Benjamin while I tried to find an after-hours line to call. While my husband walked with our son, he heard him release some gas, so he checked his diaper. We were shocked and scared when we saw his right scrotum pulsing in and out, while Benjamin continued to scream. That was enough for us, and we quickly loaded up in the car and headed to the ER.

On the way, Benjamin fell asleep. I wasn't sure if I should be relieved or concerned, but his breathing was steady, and his color was good. When we were finally taken back to a room and able to consult with a doctor, he concluded that our son's hydrocele (which had been discovered while he was in the hospital following his heart surgery) was acting up, but there was no cause for alarm as he couldn't detect a hernia. He sent us on our way and told us to keep an eye on things.

The next day I took Benjamin to a follow-up appointment with his cardiologist. His heart looked good, but he still had a trace of pulmonary hypertension, though not enough to warrant going back on medicine. I was pleased by the good report and changed Benjamin's diaper before packing up to go home. During his diaper change he cried and eventually passed a very hard stool. It occurred to me that the pain he was experiencing the night before may have been caused by constipation which triggered his hydrocele to act up. I called his pediatrician's office later in the day to get some tips on treating the constipation. However, that evening Benjamin had another episode like the night before. Something inside me told me that this may be a more serious matter than the doctor had thought, so I loaded Benjamin in the car and called Shawn, who was just getting off work, to meet me at the ER. This time a different doctor examined our son and came to the same conclusion; the constipation was activating his hydrocele, but there was no hernia. He did recommend that we follow up with our pediatrician the following week.

Over the weekend we got Benjamin's constipation under control and thankfully did not have any more episodes. On Monday I made an appointment with the pediatrician and explained to him all that had happened over the last four days. He examined Benjamin, and to my dismay said that he detected a hernia that would require outpatient surgery as soon as possible. He got us a referral to a specialist at St. Francis Children's Hospital, and we scheduled an appointment for the end of the week. Shawn's heart sunk as well when I told him the news. We were ready to enjoy the Christmas season; the last thing we wanted was to have our son in the hospital again. Why did he have to go through one more thing?

The next few days were difficult. I was hurting and angry that Benjamin was facing another surgery, though I knew this one would be minor compared to his heart surgery. I was afraid that the hernia would get worse before it could be corrected. I dreaded setting foot in a hospital again so soon. A good friend encouraged us that we had overcome the greatest hurdle with our son's heart surgery, and it was now behind us. We would make it over this smaller hurdle too. She encouraged us to offer God a sacrifice of praise in the midst of our pain. I tried to take to heart what she said and keep things in perspective, but I was so discouraged.

On one particular day that week, Benjamin was extra fussy and did not want to be put down at all. I wasn't feeling well myself, and I was so weary by the afternoon. Needing a momentary break, I went out to check the mail. Some friends of ours who had a baby boy a few months after we did had sent us a personalized Christmas card and letter, with pictures of their family and their smiling baby. I noticed that, though younger than our son, he was holding his head up with ease. Benjamin's neck was still a bit floppy, and we had to make sure he wouldn't flail his head back while being held. As I read their Christmas letter that shared about how well their son was doing and how much they were enjoying life with him (as they absolutely should), something inside of me broke. Waves of grief swept over me as I mourned the early C-section in place of a healthy, full-term delivery. I mourned the long hospital stays in the place of bringing my baby home from the start. I mourned the numerous health conditions in place of a healthy, thriving baby. I mourned the many developmental delays in the place of a typically developing child. And now we were facing another medical challenge. It wasn't fair!

I knew I was in self-pity, but I remembered the exhortation to offer a sacrifice of praise, so as I held my fussy baby, I began to sing the chorus "So Good to Me" out of sheer will. As my son's cries escalated, I sat down to nurse him, opened my Bible to Psalm 27, and began to read aloud. I didn't get very far before deep sobs rose up inside of me and I began to release my pent-up grief to the Lord. In the midst of the pain, I felt His peace wash over my heart, and I knew we weren't walking through this alone. I called my mom later and told her about the difficulties of my day. She is truly one of the best listeners I have ever known! A few days later I received the following letter from her that offered some much-needed encouragement:

Dear Dana,

We just got off the phone. I think of you, worn out from the day and relieved to have your husband home from work. I think of Shawn picking up Benjamin and saying/singing silly things to him. I think of Benjamin smiling, squawking, and screaming.

You are providing Benjamin with the best of beginnings. Giving him your attention, interacting with him, caring for his needs are precious investments. He is blessed to have you as his mommy and Shawn as his daddy.

You are wise to allow yourself to cry through the grief when it strikes and wiser yet to spend time soaking in the presence of God, the great Healer.

The easiest thing to forget and hardest thing to do for moms is to also take care of ourselves. Your grieving today is part of taking care of your emotional self. Spending time with Shawn and going on simple dates together is taking care of your relationship. Doing something you love like singing or writing a song revives your creative self.

You and Shawn are Benjamin's first impressions of God's love for him. He will be able to trust and to love and to be all of what God intends for him. You are giving him a solid foundation for his whole life.

And it isn't easy. You may feel like you don't measure up to the picture-perfect family. But believe me, to those on the outside looking in, your threesome looks pretty perfect even if you don't have the professional photos or fancy Christmas letter. What you have is far more precious: the love of Jesus poured out on your family, the wisdom of God directing your lives, and the humility and self-discipline to let God lead.

I don't have words to tell you how much I love you and Shawn and Benjamin.

Hugs,

Mom

"Sorrow carved me to the quick, so joy could fill me in the mourning."

(This sentence came to me the other day, and I thought it might mean something to you, too.)

******

The day finally arrived to meet with the specialist. His report was not what I wanted to hear. Benjamin had actually developed a *double* hernia, and he needed to have surgery very soon. It was a Friday, and his next day to perform surgeries was the following Tuesday, with a pre-op appointment scheduled for Monday. Though the procedure was typically an out-patient surgery, he wanted to admit Benjamin to the hospital to be monitored for 24 hours, considering his heart history. He assured me, however, that this was a simple surgery with an easy recovery. There would be no reason why we couldn't travel with Benjamin the following week to go to Minnesota for Christmas.

Benjamin's surgery was scheduled for first thing in the morning, which required an early check-in. Someone generously blessed us by getting us a motel room the night before, so we wouldn't have to make the hour-long drive in the wee hours of the morning. As with his heart surgery, Benjamin couldn't nurse in the morning, so he was not a happy guy as we waited for him to go back for his operation. When the time came, we weren't allowed to walk him down the hall as we had before, and I wondered if that right was reserved for the more serious surgeries or if it simply depended on the particular staff on shift. It was still difficult to see him go. The waiting room was an all too familiar sight, but Shawn and I were pleasantly surprised at how little time it took for his surgery to be completed. We received the news that everything went well, and then we were led back to the recovery area where Benjamin was waking up from anesthesia.

When we reached our small son, we encountered the most difficult part of our day. Our baby was only partially awake, but he was screaming from the disorienting effects of the anesthesia. He was too incoherent to nurse, and he seemed to be inconsolable. We knew his reaction wasn't unusual, but it was so hard to hear him cry and to feel helpless to comfort him. Shawn and I took turns passing Benjamin back and forth, and he finally fell asleep again in Shawn's arms. However, if Shawn tried to shift his position at all, our baby would cry again, so he held him in the same position for over 30 minutes, while we waited for the nurses to take us up to our hospital room. I felt bad for my husband who said his arms felt like "mush" by the end!

Once settled in to the room, Shawn headed out to go work a partial day and planned to return that evening and spend the night with us.

I spent a quiet day as Benjamin mostly slept and only woke up occasionally to nurse. I didn't have much emotional energy left and zoned out for a better part of the day watching HGTV and checking e-mail. I was thankful Benjamin's surgery went well, but it was so hard to be confined to a hospital room again, even if only for a day. Thankfully, as a nursing mom, I was still able to receive free meals delivered through room service. (This service had been a life-saver during our previous two-week stay!) If we had to be in a hospital, St. Francis Children's Hospital was the best! I was glad when Shawn returned in the evening, and we had an uneventful but fairly restless night. I slept on the narrow, built-in couch, and my poor husband slept on the cold tile floor. We were awakened every few hours while the nurses did their rounds.

Morning finally came, and now it was just the waiting game until we could be released to go home. Benjamin was doing really well; there had been no complications with the anesthesia. All of his stats looked good, and he was a happy guy, seemingly oblivious to the fact that he'd just undergone surgery. We were instructed in how to care for his surgery site over the next few weeks and assured that it looked more painful than it felt. Finally, late into the morning we were discharged.

We fell back into a rhythm fairly quickly after returning home, and we were able to drive to Minnesota and enjoy Benjamin's first Christmas without any problems. In retrospect we realized that this had indeed been only a small hurdle to cross, and, as was true with every hurdle prior, we experienced God's sustaining grace. I was reminded that more hurdles would come of all shapes and sizes (as they do in everyone's life), but the important thing is to not get side-tracked by the delays, but to keep moving forward with confidence that our God is more than able to make *"all things work together for good to those who love God, to those who are called according to His purpose,"* (Romans 8:28).

Joy in the Pain

I only logged on to check the weather. The sky looks overcast today, and I want to know how I should dress myself and Benjamin. The Internet opens to our homepage of MSN. I have no idea why that's set as our home page. Neither of us even uses Hotmail. We've just never taken the time to change it. As the pictures come into view, a particular one catches my eye—a peaceful, sleeping newborn curled up in a basket of sorts. It reminds me of an Anne Geddes pose, though this article is highlighting a sister photography duo. There's a link to view twenty-four pictures of sleeping babies. I can't help myself and open it up, calling for Shawn to come and see. We "ooh" and "aah" over the adorable photos of newborns asleep in baskets, buckets, sarongs, or cradled in hands. I even open the short video interviewing the twin photographers as they discuss their strategies for capturing such unbelievable poses. They also discuss their new book, something about babies in a dreamland. The pictures seem like windows into another world, a world in which everything is peace, safety, and pure happiness. The video even highlights one set of customers, who so wanted to capture the first sweet moments with their newborn, they drove an extra distance to the photographers' studio to let the sisters work their magic.

I finally navigate away from the page to check what I really intended to see. The forecast today gives a high of 66 degrees with possible rain. I log off the Internet and get ready for my shower, thoughts tumbling through my head. The pictures made me smile; I couldn't help myself in the face of such pure adorableness. Viewing the photos brought a tinge of pain as well, though. I can't help but think of my own newborn pictures of Benjamin, all in the NICU, with his array of tubes and wires while a ventilator did most of his breathing for him. Like the pictures of the sleeping babies he, too, was asleep, though his was a sedated, unnatural sleep.

Instead of the pink, healthy newborn skin his was gray and ashy, followed by a yellowed tint as jaundice set in, and redness as his belly swelled bigger and bigger due to kidney failure. Instead of pictures of a baby sleeping peacefully in the parents' arms, our pictures show us touching little hands in the NICU bed, our only contact with our son for the first nine days of his life. At the time I write this, none of the pictures are yet printed. They are all still saved on the digital camera and computer. They are not the sort of photos to frame and proudly display on a wall or bookshelf. They are shots that speak of uncertainty, helplessness and pain—not the joy of a new arrival.

The thoughts and words I am now writing flow through my mind as the warm water of the shower flows over my body. As I think and remember, though, an important realization comes to mind. The babies pictured in "dreamland" may appear to come from perfect families in perfect homes with perfect lives, but I know this is not the case. It can never be the case, for no family is perfect, and no life is immune from pain and troubles. I find myself wondering what the stories behind these beautiful babies might be. What is life like in their families? What unique struggles have they had to face? Most importantly, do they know the One who can sustain them through those struggles? I have experienced pain, but I have a Friend who's walked with me every step of the way. I have cried many tears, but I have a Comforter who's caught each and every one in a bottle and considered them precious. I have had many questions, but I have a Counselor who speaks peace to my heart, even when I don't understand. I have felt helpless and afraid, but I have a Father who's wrapped me in His embrace and assured me of His love and protection. Yes, I have had pain…but I know the One who enables me to discover joy in the midst of the pain. I pray that through our story others may find Him as well.

God's Formula

His beautiful eyes stare into mine as the milk begins to flow. Those big blue eyes with the delicate Brushfield spots gaze at me with trust and adoration. In between gulps he pulls back just to smile and coo. Warm milk drips down my skin, but I don't mind. My baby just smiled at me. He lifts his chubby hand to my mouth, waiting expectantly for my kisses. If I don't respond quickly enough, he grabs hold of my lip, eyes locked onto my own. At almost eleven months and nearly 24 pounds, this is still his favorite part of the day: mine, too. The bond that we share is precious, and I wouldn't give it up for anything.

Some family and friends are surprised that I'm still breastfeeding, and they certainly can't imagine me nursing Benjamin past his first birthday. Over the months I've heard the subtle comments such as "Oh, you're still nursing?" or "How long do you intend to breastfeed?" or "When he goes on the bottle…" What they don't realize is that he's not going on the bottle. I want to give my son the best start I can, nutritionally, relationally, and developmentally. My milk is "God's formula" as our wonderful pediatrician loves to say. Benjamin is learning to trust and to love at my breast. His tongue and jaws are gaining strength as he pulls the milk from me, all preparing his muscles for future speech.

My mother nursed my brother and me into our toddler years. I think we are the better for it. I dreamed all my life of nursing my babies. I've had to fight hard to fulfill this dream, harder than I ever imagined. I am going to cherish this time.

There was the month of pumping in the NICU. The lactation consultant taught me how to hook up, operate, and clean the Medela breast pump and attachments. It was the hospital grade pump and, as she described it, the "Lexus" of all breast pumps. My emotions swung back and forth between gratitude for this device that enabled me to build and maintain my milk supply and resentment for the sterile, mechanical hum of a machine in the place of my baby. There was the exhaustion of pumping every three hours around the clock while recovering from a C-section, coupled with the emotional wounds that were always bleeding. There was the constant bottle of water on hand—drinking, drinking, drinking. There was the ravenous appetite as more and more calories went into milk production. There was the thrill of watching the small bottles slowly filling fuller and fuller as the days went by and my supply was built up. There was the bittersweetness of seeing my milk fed to my son through a feeding tube straight into his stomach; tiny amounts at first as his tiny system adjusted. At least he was receiving nourishment from my body. There were the first few failed attempts at nursing and the slow process of learning to bottle feed with the therapist. *Breathe, suck, swallow.* There was the devastation of hearing that the NICU had run out of my milk one night and had to supplement Benjamin with formula. My milk was one of the only things I had a measure of control over; one of the only things I could give to my son at that point. I cried, feeling I had failed him. My resolve to persevere with the pumping was strengthened even more. There were the constant nagging fears that Benjamin might never breastfeed, as medical professionals reminded me of his low muscle tone and possible poor sucking reflex common in babies with Down syndrome. There was the first precious time Benjamin latched on for a moment and looked up at me with wonder and confusion in this little face. *How many ways are there for me to eat?* I could almost hear him thinking.

Then we were finally home, and there was the nipple shield to enable him to latch on. There was the struggle of holding his floppy neck steady, directing him to my breast as he rooted around, and holding the nipple shield in place. All too soon there was the second trip to the hospital for open heart surgery and the extended two week stay. Once again there was the rhythmic humming of the "Lexus" pump around the clock. Once again there was the stress, the exhaustion, and the fear I wouldn't be able to maintain my supply. This time there was a heightened physical ache to hold my son close to my breast again and feel the sweet release.

A few weeks later there was the second home-coming and the supplementing with bottles of milk I had already pumped while I built up my supply again. In time there were the first few awkward experiences of breastfeeding in public with my special nursing cover, complicated by the use of the nipple shield. Eventually there was the long process of weaning Benjamin from the nipple shield. When he was in a calm mood, he could latch on to my right side without the shield with some patience and coaxing. The left side seemed to create more problems. If he was in a fussy mood, he would fight and scream until I gave in and put the shield back in place. There was the excitement when he was finally able to latch on to both sides and the relief when the nipple shield was put away for good.

Today, Benjamin is a pro at nursing. He quickly latches on without my assistance, eager for the warmth and comfort of Mommy's breast. The milk is paying off too. His arms and legs consist of delightful rolls, his tummy is big and round, and his cheeks are so plump and kissable. Strangers comment on what a cute and healthy baby he is. *Healthy*--that word is so special to hear. I doubt that they would ever guess the premature birth or the ventilator, tubes, and wires. They know nothing of the jaundice, the bloated stomach when his kidneys shut down, or the home-coming with nose cannulas and oxygen tanks. They would never imagine the open heart surgery and slow recovery. They have no idea about the ER visits leading to the discovery of double hernias and the following surgery. They are oblivious to the onset of seizures, infantile spasms to be exact, and the six week treatment of shots. Failed hearing tests and ear tube surgery never crosses their minds. (More on all that later.) They simply see a beautiful, healthy, baby boy…which he is…my little miracle.

Memories and Miracles

I'm trying to catch fifteen extra minutes of shut eye after our morning nursing session. Benjamin is sitting happily in his baby seat in the office with Daddy. As I lie in bed, sleep eludes me while memories sweep through my mind at a rapid rate. For no rhyme or reason I am escorted back to May 2009. I remember the unexpected and frightening C-section, the first piercing cries of my newborn son, and the shock and fear when he was rushed to the NICU instead of being brought to me. I remember my first glimpse of my baby four hours later, hooked up to a ventilator and monitors, his skin an unnatural ashy color. The doctor had already told us she suspected Down syndrome and kept saying, "He's a very sick little boy." I remember when I finally got to hold my son nine days later, though he was still a tangle of tubes and wires. I remember the day of his longed-for homecoming when he was a month old, and the nurse's parting comment, "He truly is a miracle. Most of us didn't expect him to still be here." I remember the short-lived month at home before Benjamin was back in the hospital for open heart surgery and a two week recovery in the PICU…

…My memories are interrupted by the obnoxious beeping of my alarm clock, and I tell myself that it really is time to get up and start the day. I walk into the office and kneel down beside my beautiful 16-month old miracle to give him kisses. His face lights up in a huge grin. "Hello, Miracle Man!" I say as I pick him up and hold him close. Benjamin lets out a delighted squeal. We head to the living room for him to play with his favorite toys—a Leap Frog Learn & Groove Musical Table and a highlighter-yellow stuffed gorilla. As I sip my coffee and watch my son eagerly playing, I am struck with the beautiful thought that every day with Benjamin is truly a miracle!

Journey

Spring 1984—Mom watched Randy after school until his parents got off work. The bus would drop him off at our little townhouse where he would spend the next few hours. Randy was a teenager with dark hair and a stocky build. Randy loved to eat the food Mom fixed for him. One day while savoring his third helping of a dish he particularly enjoyed, he was curious to know the ingredients. When Mom mentioned "peanut butter" his eyes grew wide and much to Mom's exasperation he exclaimed, "I can't eat anymore. I don't like peanut butter!"

One of Randy's favorite pastimes when he visited us was to look through Mom's jewelry box. She would set it out for him, and one by one he would study each piece with great care and wonder. He was able to take pleasure in simple things.

Randy was my buddy. Though he was sixteen and I was barely two we had a wonderful time together. I would sit on his lap and we would count together…one, two, three…Randy had a hard time getting past three, but it didn't seem to bother him when I would count up to ten. It didn't bother me, either. Randy was my friend, and I looked up to him because he was older than me. I didn't know that Randy had Down syndrome; I didn't even know what Down syndrome was. I knew that Randy was nice and fun, and I loved it when he came over to play…I have no personal memories of Randy; they were lost somewhere back in the early years of childhood. I remember Mom's stories, though, and I remember a snapshot of me sitting in my friend's lap, an unlikely but happy duo.

******

1995—Michael's family only attended our church for a few years. His parents were an older couple who could have just as easily passed as his grandparents. Michael was just a little boy, old enough to walk but not yet in school. I watched him in the nursery on occasion with some of the other children. As a young teen who loved kids, I looked forward to nursery duty. My most vivid memories of Michael are his big brown eyes and contagious smile. I knew Michael had Down syndrome but didn't have any clear ideas about what that meant. I knew he was a bit slower than other children and looked a bit different than they did, but I just treated him the same as everyone else. He was a little boy, and he was adorable!

******

2000-2004—My college years. Emily worked in the cafeteria on campus. She was very short, and so I was surprised to learn she was actually a few years older than me. She worked hard, staying focused and task-oriented. If someone she was not acquainted with approached her, Emily would fold her arms, narrow her eyes and ask "Do I know you?" Emily loved the movie *Grease* so much that her family gave her a specially made "Pink Ladies" jacket, which she proudly sported around the campus. Emily's dad was a religion professor for the university and was a favorite of his students. Emily had her daddy wrapped around her little finger in a good way. One cell phone call from her would interrupt any class at any time. Sometimes she just called to say hi, but sometimes she called to let her daddy know her blood sugar was too high or too low, and he would drop everything to rush home and check on her, not wanting to take any chances with her diabetic condition. His love for his daughter was so apparent and touching. My knowledge of Down syndrome was still next to nothing. I knew I had heard somewhere that people with Down syndrome had shortened life spans, and I felt sad for the professor and his family, wondering how long they would have with Emily. My information was outdated at best.

December 2008—We were in Minnesota with my husband's family for the holidays. I was just entering the second trimester of my first pregnancy, eager to show off the beginning of my "baby bump." Shawn and I were ecstatic and knew I carried the perfect child inside of me. During a Christmas celebration with my father-in-law's side of the family, I met Clint. Clint was my age and was the brother-in-law of one of Shawn's cousins. He occasionally came along for family gatherings with the Hemmingers, though this was my first time to meet him. Shawn had become acquainted with him several years before at a graduation event. He remembered Clint's name and was intentional to introduce us. Though Clint's speech was difficult to understand, we tried to make friendly conversation with him. As the day carried on I noticed that, for the most part, he stayed close to his young niece and nephew or sat by himself. However, Clint was very friendly and happy to talk when someone else made the initiative, so I found myself building a puzzle on the floor with the kids and engaging with him in conversation. Obviously touched by the fact that my husband had remembered his name and shown him kindness at their first meeting and again that day, Clint went on and on about how nice Shawn was and how much he liked him. He told me a bit about his group home and about his girlfriend, a topic he was very proud of! Though I'm sure I missed a lot of what he said due to his unclear speech, I was happy to have a chance to be a listening ear and to show him kindness. I would not be entirely honest, however, if I did not admit that I experienced some discomfort as well. I still knew so little about Down syndrome, and some of Clint's behaviors and mannerisms were awkward to me. Though I wanted to show love to him, at times I would find myself looking for a way to excuse myself from further conversation, at least for a while.

March 2009—Our prayer group was hosting a special speaker from out of town. The woman had her children with her, one of whom was an elementary school-aged girl with an extra chromosome. That night a testimony was given from a member of our group, who was a long- time friend of the speaker, about how much she had experienced God's love through this little girl's affection. After the meeting the little girl came up to me, staring intently at my rounded belly. She stretched out her hand, touched me and exclaimed "Fat!" before walking away. She repeated this a second time before the night was over. I laughed at her boldness and her innocence. However, seeing this little girl made me think of the blood test just a few months prior that indicated I may be carrying a child with Down syndrome. When the baby's measurements appeared normal in the ultrasound, we were convinced the blood test had been a false-positive reading. I was so relieved.

******

May 2, 2009—The chapel at the university was packed and overflowing as people filled the seats for the upcoming graduation ceremony. Shawn was out of town for a few days at a men's camp, so I attended alone on behalf of both of us to see our friend receive his degree. Big, pregnant, and extremely uncomfortable, I wondered if anyone would recognize my plight and offer me a seat. I finally found favor next to some acquaintances from the university and settled my tired body into the cushioned seat. As I watched the crowd around me, I noticed Emily running up the steps of the chapel in the direction of the bathroom. Her father, wearing his official graduation attire, sat on the stage with the other professors and administrators, keeping a watchful eye on his daughter, even from a distance. I wondered what life had been like for him, his wife, and their other children. My mind wandered back to January, and the brief scare that our baby would have Down syndrome. I felt my son kick inside me, and felt relieved again that I hadn't been asked to walk that road.

******

May 22, 2009—Benjamin Lee Hemminger was born with an extra chromosome and numerous complications. I suddenly found myself thrust onto a road I didn't want to walk, a road that appeared so dark and uncertain. Every step was shaky, and I had no sense of direction. The only thing that was certain was that this was my son, and I loved him no matter what.

******

September 26, 2010—I have been on this road one year, four months, and four days. The darkness of those early days has lifted, though there are still many steps that feel uncertain. The incredible love and joy I have in my heart for my son gives me direction, however, and the love of my Heavenly Father steadies my steps. I am privileged to be Benjamin's mother, and it is my delight to love him. As I have reminisced today, I have realized that my journey with Benjamin began before I ever knew I was on a journey. Even as a two year old in Randy's lap, the egg that would join my husband's seed to conceive our beautiful son was within me. In a small way Benjamin was already a part of me and has always been a part of me. In His wisdom and sovereignty, God gave me opportunities throughout my early life to see *individuals* with Down syndrome, though I did not recognize the significance of these encounters at the time. I am so grateful that He knows every step of my journey--past, present, and future--and that He lovingly gives me sign-posts along the way. It is a journey I never expected, a journey I would not have requested, but it is a journey I will cherish every day.

Sacrifice of Praise

Psalm 116:17 reads *"I will offer to You the sacrifice of thanksgiving and will call on the name of the Lord."* One of the hardest things to do when you're hurting is to praise God. It doesn't come naturally. It takes a determined act of the will. And when you're really hurting, it's hard to find the determination to do much of anything.

I wrestled with this over and over in the months following my son's birth. I didn't want to praise God; I was angry with God, and I would feel guilty for my anger one moment and justified in it the next. At the same time, though, I knew I couldn't survive without Jesus, and the fear of my heart growing cold towards Him was greater than the anger in my heart. So, I would pour out my emotions to Him and ask Him to heal my heart. But to *praise* Him, to *thank* Him in the midst of so much heartbreak, was a constant struggle.

However, as time went on and I *chose* to praise Him, even though I was torn and bleeding and didn't *feel* like praising Him, my heart slowly started to come alive again. I discovered that there can truly be joy in the midst of sorrow. I also realized that it was and is a privilege to praise Jesus in the midst of my pain, for this is a gift I can only bring to Him during this short season of earthly time. Life passes by like a mist and then eternity is upon us. For those who have been born again by the sacrificial blood of Jesus, He promises to *"...wipe away every tear from their eyes,"* in the age to come (see Revelation 7:17). In this tiny window of opportunity, I can give Him the gift of my love and my worship in the middle of my pain. What a precious thing to bring to the One who endured so much pain and suffering for me because of love!

I play guitar and have been writing songs since 2005. Sitting with my guitar before the Lord and singing to Him in worship is such a big part of who I am. However, for months after Benjamin's birth, my guitar sat untouched. For a season I stepped down from leading worship at my church and at our prayer group gatherings. It just wasn't in me. I knew healing was beginning to take place inside when I started to pick up my guitar again. However pre-written songs couldn't express what was in my heart, so I sat down with pen and paper one day and wrote lyrics for a new song to the Lord, which is as much to say that I wrote out a prayer. In a short time, the Holy Spirit gave me music to go with the words, and I was once again able to express my heart before Him in song. What a release and freedom came as a result! From the place of praise and worship, life's cares take on their proper perspective, and I am reminded that I am created for Him and Him alone. My life is to be lived unto His glory, and He can do whatever He wants with me. He is perfect love and perfect peace, and He is orchestrating things for my best interest from an *eternal perspective.* One day in eternity, I will look back and see the wisdom and beauty of His leadership over my life, and, oh, how I will praise Him in that day!

For I know the thoughts that I think toward you, says the Lord, thoughts of peace and not of evil, to give you a future and a hope. Then you will call upon Me and go and pray to Me, and I will listen to you. And you will seek Me and find Me when you search for Me with all your heart, (Jeremiah 29:11-13).

<u>Awakening</u> (my song)

Why does my heart feel so numb?

Where has the fire gone?

I slumber and I stumble in the dark of night.

When will I see the dawn?

I remember the rainbows after the rain,

Your promises spoken to me.

So I stir up my soul and I cry out to You

The One who holds the key

More than answers, I want Your face.

More than solutions, I need Your embrace

So I lay down my heart, Lord, down at Your feet

To be broken, awakened, healed, and set free.

I want what's real, what's fresh and alive.

This is my heart's deepest cry.

Weed out the doubt, lies, and confusion.

Cause this flesh to die.

Make my life a prelude to heaven,

Completely consumed by You.

Holy Spirit, come and fan the flame,

You who make all things new.

More than answers, I want Your face.

More than solutions, I need Your embrace,

So I lay down my heart, Lord, down at Your feet

To be broken, awakened, healed, and set free.

Eyes of the Beholder

"Are you okay? I know they look kind of Mr. Magooish," said the lady at the eye glasses center after fitting Benjamin's new glasses for the first time. I winced at the association; with their thick, round, bright blue frames, her description was right on the mark. A few months prior, Benjamin had eye surgery to correct the strabismus--a condition that causes the eyes to cross--in both eyes. The surgery had been mostly successful but had not completely fixed the problem. His eye doctor recommended glasses to give him the added assistance needed to correctly focus, assuring me that Benjamin would probably outgrow the need for them by his twelfth birthday. Even with this knowledge, I felt such a resistance rise up inside of me, not wanting to accept that this would be my son's new "look." How would people see his beautiful blue eyes or his sweeping, long eyelashes that were so often commented on? Sadly, I began to assume the worst. Instead of the endearing stares of others, I pictured people looking on with disdain at the poor child who obviously has "problems." Thirty minutes later at my favorite sandwich shop I was given the chance to test my theory. While standing in line I noticed a woman staring at us, and I immediately became protective on the inside. A few minutes later, however, she approached me to share that she had glasses from the time she was a small child and asked a few disarming questions about Benjamin. Later a staff member stopped to talk to Benjamin, ask some questions, and tell him how handsome he was with his new glasses. On the way out of the restaurant, two teenage girls giggled and smiled with adoration as we passed by. So much for my theory...

This was not the first (and probably won't be the last) time insecurity has gripped me in regards to my son's appearance. During those first shaky weeks in the NICU following his birth, I tried to comprehend what his diagnosis of Down syndrome would mean. It sounds shallow, I know, and I almost felt guilty for thinking it, but one of my concerns was what he would look like to other people. All through my pregnancy I daydreamed about the perfect calendar baby (what parent doesn't), whose face could grace the front of any greeting card. The stark reality of having a child with a disability caused me to ask the question, "Will anyone but our own family think he's beautiful?" Time and again, though, I was proven wrong as complete strangers would stop me in stores, restaurants, and doctor's offices just to take a closer look at my "adorable" baby. In the first few months my thought was, "They must not realize that he has Down syndrome." As my acceptance of his diagnosis has unfolded, though, I've thought that less and less. Benjamin is beautiful as Benjamin, 47 chromosomes and all!

Just after my son's first birthday, he was fitted with hearing aids in both ears. *(I will share about this in greater detail later on)*. Since you can't hide a hearing aid, we decided to have fun with the ear mold color and chose a soft blue. "Maybe it will bring out his eyes," I reasoned with myself. Once again, though, insecurity took hold, and my emotions resisted this new "look" for my son. I grieved inside, thinking the days of people commenting on my beautiful baby were over. "He'll get stares, but it will be for a different reason now." I was sure of it. Once again I was proven wrong, though, as Benjamin continued to have a magnetic pull that drew people to him. In time I grew accustomed to the hearing aids, and they have just become a normal part of life. We even decorate the hearing aids themselves with specialty stickers. Our sticker of choice is a pair of lions, continuing his nursery theme.

It is early January 2011 as I write this, and Benjamin has had the glasses for a few weeks now. I can't say that I'm fully adjusted to them yet, but the sting is dissolving. Some of my concerns have been proven true as far as the difficulty of keeping glasses on a baby and keeping them clean, but other concerns have been blown out of the water. We recently attended the 2010 One Thing Conference at the International House of Prayer in Kansas City, and Shawn and I were overwhelmed by the response Benjamin received from others. We could barely go ten minutes without someone walking by and smiling or stopping to talk to Benjamin. I can't remember how many times someone would come up just to say "Excuse me, but your son is so adorable!" One young lady stopped in the middle of a crowd just to stare and had others run into her! People were simply drawn to Benjamin left and right.

Now, I'm tempted to say it's because my son really is that exceptionally cute (which in my mind he absolutely is!), but I think it goes deeper than that. The world is full of cute babies, but Benjamin seems to carry something special. There is a peace and a joy that rests on him, and I know it is by the Holy Spirit. People who see him seem to have an automatic love and affection for him, and he imparts joy to so many. We have heard time and time again since his birth, "Benjamin is such a blessing!" His presence in a room seems to affect the atmosphere around him, and everyone who comes in contact with him leaves with a smile on their face. That is not something Shawn or I can take credit for; I know that it is the Lord in him. God's beauty rests upon Benjamin, and it is contagious!

I've heard it said that "beauty is in the eyes of the beholder," and I've also heard it said that "you become what you behold." As much as it warms my heart to see Benjamin fawned over by others, I realize how much needless energy I've wasted on worrying about what other people think. Even if my fears had materialized and people looked on my son with disdain, it would not change Benjamin's beauty. His Heavenly Father and Creator crafted Benjamin in His image, and He only creates masterpieces. The only gaze that truly matters is the passionate gaze of my loving King, and I know that as I behold Him, I will be transformed more and more into His beautiful likeness. I want to teach my son to live before an "audience of One," finding his confidence and identity in the reality of how God sees him. I want him to live as one who continues to impart joy and hope to others because of Whose Presence he abides in. I want him to be one who can see the beauty in all people, viewing them through heaven's perspective. The things I want for my son, I must model. I know that as I set my heart to gaze on Jesus and His beauty, He will empower me to do so.

On a side note, in His goodness, God let me experience having a calendar baby! In the 2011 Down Syndrome Association of Tulsa (DSAT) calendar, Benjamin and his daddy proudly share the spotlight with two other father/child duos for the month of June. The theme for the month is "Dads as heroes." I'm so thankful Benjamin has a Daddy whose hero is his Heavenly Father, whose eyes behold the beauty of his God, and who will teach our son to do the same!

Postscript:

As it turned out, Benjamin had a second eye surgery the following August that made a big improvement in the strabismus, eliminating his need for glasses. A third surgery was required again in the fall of 2013, and it was very successful. While the season with glasses was short-lived, I hope the lessons learned will be life-long. Benjamin has continued to grace DSAT calendars with his joyful smile!

Touching Millions

"Your son will encourage millions." These words were spoken by a complete stranger as Shawn pushed Benjamin around in his stroller at the back of the huge conference hall at the Kansas City Convention Center. We were attending the 2010 One Thing Conference hosted by the International House of Prayer (IHOP) in Kansas City, MO. At least 22,000 people, mostly youth and young adults had gathered for four days of seeking after the heart of Jesus as we prepared to celebrate the start of a new year. Millions more were tuning in by TV or Internet connections from around the world. Shawn thanked the man and came to find me so he could share what had just happened. I quickly recorded the words of encouragement in my journal. A few hours later I received a text message from the (IHOP) testimony team, asking if we would be willing to share our son's testimony on the stage that night, which happened to be New Year's Eve and the last night of the conference. His testimony...I'd better do some backtracking...

In January 2010 I began to notice some strange behavior in Benjamin. At random times, though usually after waking up, his eyes would get a distant look, his shoulders would hunch up, and his arms would spread out to the sides a bit. He would repeat this motion multiple times within a few minute timeframe. Whatever he had been engaged in would be momentarily interrupted. I noticed it first while nursing him. He would lose his latch for a few moments and then resume again. After about a week of noticing this behavior on and off, I called it to Shawn's attention. Alarmed, he asked me to get an appointment with the pediatrician the next week. Neither of us wanted to say "seizures," but a haunting fear was beginning to grow in us. I felt guilty for not saying something sooner. I had tried so hard to convince myself that it was nothing; maybe he was just passing gas or a little constipated. I didn't think I could handle another medical challenge for my little eight month old baby. Benjamin had just had surgery the month prior to fix the double hernias in his groin area. In some ways we were still recovering from his open heart surgery the previous July.

When we saw Dr. Harris a few days later, he wasted no time in referring us to a pediatric neurologist. However, as is often the case with specialists, the office was booked for six weeks and gave us no hope of getting in any sooner. As we anxiously waited for his appointment, Benjamin's condition grew worse. The episodes became more and more frequent, averaging two to four "clusters" a day, whereas before we only noticed one or two every few days or so. Developmentally he began to take steps backwards. His smile and laugh, which had only just been emerging, disappeared altogether. He would no longer make eye contact with Mommy or Daddy. He was not interested in playing with toys or playing in general. He spent a lot of time just laying around and staring into space.

The day of his appointment finally arrived, but instead of seeing a specialist, we saw a technician who performed an EEG. Benjamin was wrapped up like a burrito, then had numerous leads and wires attached to his head (a long process). Once everything was in place, the lights were turned off, except for occasional flashing lights over Benjamin, and his brain activity was charted on the computer for twenty minutes. My heart sank when I realized the technician could not give me any information about what the computer was reading; we would have to wait for the neurologist to read the results and call them in to our doctor's office. Two long weeks later our pediatrician called asking me to bring Benjamin in right away. My mom was visiting at the time and was with me as Dr. Harris shared the news. He had just received the EEG results that morning. The test showed chaotic brain activity, indicating a form of seizures known as infantile spasms, a condition more common in children with Down syndrome. Without missing a beat he personally called the neurologist's office, insisting that Benjamin be seen within a few days. We had an appointment scheduled for two days later. After receiving the news in the doctor's office, I felt numb. Thank God for my mom who had the presence of mind to ask more questions and write some things down so we could begin our own research. We went straight to Shawn's office so I could personally tell him what we'd discovered. Upon hearing the news, he broke down crying. My tears wouldn't come until later; I was still numb and in a state of denial.

The next few days brought more discouragement as we found more information about infantile spasms. There was no fool-proof treatment for the condition. It carried the potential of long-term brain damage and increased developmental delay. There was a chance of the development of other types of seizures down the road. Our appointment with the neurologist didn't brighten things either. He explained to us that there were different types of medications to try, but all of them had potential (and some severe) side effects, and none of them were guaranteed to solve the problem. At best they could stop the seizure activity, though there would still be the potential of future onset; at worst they wouldn't do anything for the seizures and Benjamin could experience side effects. His first recommendation for treatment was called ACTH (abbreviated), and would require six weeks of shots—three weeks of daily injections and three weeks of every other day. He told us the pediatrician's office could teach us to administer them. *Give my baby shots?!* I'd never imagined having to do such a thing, but do it we must.

The first week of treatment saw us daily at the doctor's office. I was the first to try administering the shot, and I could think of a million other things I'd rather be doing. To have to intentionally inflict pain on my child felt like more than I could bear. Shawn was in an even worse state. The day he had to give the shot he almost passed out. He was so shaken he asked me to pray for him before he left. I found out later, to my slight irritation, that he even stopped to get himself ice cream on the way back to work to help him feel better, while I went to another part of the hospital to get Benjamin's daily blood pressure reading. (Yes, I have forgiven him!) As it was, I ended up administering all the rest of the treatments.

The week uncovered more concerns as well. Benjamin's glucose levels were tested before the first shot was administered, and were slightly high. This pattern continued throughout the first week. Now in addition to giving him shots, we had to prick his toe on a regular basis to test his blood sugar levels. During this *same* week, Benjamin failed a hearing test which started the ball rolling for a long series of events that culminated with him being fitted for hearing aids a few months later. He had to have extra lab work that week as well, and he is very much a "hard stick." He wailed inconsolably while being poked and prodded like a pin cushion before they could finally draw blood.

Our mountain of troubles seemed to be rising higher and higher at an alarming rate. Emotionally I was hanging by a thread. I tried to hold on to the words of encouragement the Lord had spoken to me while I was waiting on Him a few days before we received the confirmation of our son's seizures. I had a dream that it was my fault Benjamin had Down syndrome. When I told Shawn my dream, he encouraged me to take time to ask God for the truth that would displace this lie in my mind and emotions. I did so and was amazed at the words I felt the Holy Spirit speak straight into my heart:

I have chosen Benjamin for Myself, and I will release My glory through him. His condition is not a tragedy but an opportunity for Me to show Myself strong. Do not grow weary and do not lose heart, for I have chosen your family for such a time as this. I will yet wipe every tear from your eyes and restore joy where there has been sorrow. I AM God, and I will do this, so look to Me. Always look to Me.

During the first week of shots, Benjamin was understandably more fussy than usual. There were afternoons that he would just scream and scream, behavior that had been pretty uncharacteristic for him before. Drawing up the shots was nerve-wracking. The solution was thick and had to be refrigerated. I had to warm up the vial in my hands until the ACTH was fluid enough to be drawn out. All air bubbles had to be tapped out of the syringe before the shot could be administered, which often took a long time. Benjamin's legs were soon covered with little red spots where the multiple injections had been given. My eyes were often red with tears.

At the beginning of the second week, we finally had the Internet hooked up in our home. As a stay-at-home mom, I needed a link to the outside world. I immediately went to the International House of Prayer website, which streams the 24/7 worship and prayer that has been continuing unbroken since 1999. Benjamin loves music, especially worship music, and I needed something to help me refocus and connect with God. IHOP was also in the middle of revival, holding Awakening services several evenings a week. Testimonies were pouring in from around the world of people receiving salvation as well as physical and emotional healing. During the first day that I had the prayer room playing in the background, I noticed that Benjamin was much calmer than he had been since starting his treatments. He didn't have a single screaming fit that day. The next day he was lying on his baby gym mat in the living room, and I was doing something in the kitchen. Suddenly, I heard him let out a delighted squeal. I ran into the living room and saw what my heart had been aching to see for months. Benjamin smiled big, let out another happy squeal and drifted into a peaceful sleep. The next few days brought more improvements. He began reaching for toys and was even setting off musical toys he'd never been able to activate before. He was smiling, babbling, and reaching for our faces. *He did not have a single seizure that week. He has not had a single seizure since.*

By the end of the week I could hardly contain my excitement, and I e-mailed our story to IHOP. The next evening, a friend called and asked "Are you watching the Awakening service tonight? They just read your letter!" We logged onto the archives the next day and watched as Wes Hall, who was leading the service, read excerpts of our testimony that had "so touched [his] heart." In his crisp, British accent he said he believed Benjamin's testimony was a "down payment" of what God wants to do in our son and in the Down syndrome community. We were thrilled!

The next week, Benjamin's child development specialist came for our weekly in home therapy appointment. She was so shocked and thrilled by the drastic improvements in him that she stayed an extra hour. He was very engaged in the activities of the session. At one point she exclaimed, "It's amazing what a difference a week can make!" I responded, "It's amazing what a difference Jesus can make!" She agreed.

As God's timing would have it, our prayer group had already been planning a trip up to IHOP that weekend. While we were there, we had the opportunity to share Benjamin's testimony on stage, and many people prayed over him, including a young man who had been previously healed of seizures himself. During our visit, I also received some deep emotional healing. One evening some family friends offered to keep an eye on Benjamin during the service so Shawn and I could be free to go up to the front to worship and pray without distraction. Shortly after, a lady who knew our friends came up to me and asked if she could pray with me. She sensed that God wanted to heal some deep disappointments in my heart. I let her pray, but I was feeling pretty good emotionally at that point. However, as the Holy Spirit began to minister to my heart, He unplugged a well inside me, and I found myself sobbing in this woman's arms. All I could say was, "Why my son? Why my son?" As I allowed the grief to pour out, I felt lighter and freer to worship. Before the evening was over, God had touched my heart in a powerful way as wave after wave of His peace swept over me. It was a definite turning point in my journey of healing.

We dutifully finished out the course of the shots, but the amazing thing was that during and after our time at IHOP, Benjamin didn't cry during a single injection. The follow-up EEG showed that his brain waves were completely free of seizure activity! While I know that medicine is often a gift from God, I don't attribute Benjamin's amazing recovery to the medicine but to the power of the Holy Spirit. Nothing else could explain the sudden change and turn around in his condition and behaviors. At a six month EEG check-up Benjamin continued to show no sign of seizure activity. He has truly been healed!

Now we'll get back to the 2010 One Thing Conference. During our second day there, "by chance" we ran into Wes Hall and reminded him of Benjamin and his story. Wes was excited to see us and prayed over Benjamin again. On our last day, I filled out a testimony sheet for something the Lord had done for me during the conference and mentioned Benjamin's previous healing. Those things taken together prompted the testimony team to request that we share our son's story again, along with some others who would be testifying about their recent healings. As we waited backstage to go on that night, I realized that millions would be watching. I suddenly remembered the word spoken to us by a stranger only that afternoon. "Your son will encourage millions." My heart was overwhelmed as I realized God was already fulfilling that word to one degree! After we shared our testimony, Wes prayed over

Benjamin again, and we returned to our seats. As the evening came to a close, we were amazed by how many people approached us, some with tears in their eyes to thank us for sharing our son's story. Several asked if they could pray for him right then and there. We felt absolutely blanketed in God's love! My heart was warmed as well to consider the many stories we may never hear this side of eternity, of lives that were touched that night by the testimony of God's faithfulness to Benjamin!

A Day at the Park

The weather has been truly beautiful today. The temperature is in the mid 70's, the sun is shining, and there is a gentle breeze—I had to take Benjamin outside. I considered a simple walk around the neighborhood, but it just didn't seem appealing today. I considered laying a blanket out on the front lawn and blowing bubbles, but I really wanted to be able to move around more. Then I considered Johnstone Park. It seemed to be the right fit for such a beautiful day. Nestled on the outskirts of downtown Bartlesville with the Caney River looping around it, Johnstone Park offers both beautiful trees and wide open spaces, a lovely walking trail, covered picnic areas and playground equipment. So, after our afternoon nursing session I packed up a small diaper bag, and we loaded up in the car.

As I had anticipated, the park was full of activity. The playground area was swarming with children, mostly from the Boys and Girls Club who are out of school for spring break. Vehicles dotted the parking areas. I pulled in next to a pick-up truck where two elderly men sat with the windows down, leisurely conversing. After getting Benjamin situated in his stroller, I headed for the walking trail. I was thankful that the path itself looked pretty empty; most of the activity was in the playground area. As we walked I breathed in the fresh air, enjoyed the surroundings, and took time to quietly pray and reflect.

During Benjamin's first few days of life, our friend Myong went jogging at Johnstone Park daily, praying and crying out to God for Benjamin's life. Months after he was born she revealed to us that after seeing our son for the first time, she held back her tears until she left us, wondering how in the world he could survive. As she jogged and prayed over those few days, God used simple things in nature such as four-leaf clovers and butterflies and birds to speak to her about His hand over Benjamin's life. It was a sweet realization that I was now walking with my beautiful son on the same path where Myong had spent so much time praying for him to live.

At one point we stopped to sit at a bench. I had Benjamin face me in his stroller, and we played his favorite clapping game (discovered by Grandma Jan) where I clap my hands, and he places his hand in between mine. I gave him kisses, and he squealed and grabbed for my face before we resumed our walk. We soon came to the end of the path, but I didn't feel ready to go home yet. I looked over to the playground area that was such a buzz of activity and wrestled with whether or not to take Benjamin to the toddler equipment. As he is not even crawling yet, I knew there wouldn't be much we could do, but I thought he might at least be able to go down a slide with Mommy holding him.

The toddler gym was mostly empty except for one or two children. One little boy was giggling and running all over the gym as a woman (whether his mother or grandmother, I'm not sure) pretended to chase after him. She smiled at me and then watched as I held Benjamin and tried to familiarize him with some of the equipment. I then held him up to a slide and tried to help him slide down. Not knowing what to think of this new experience, Benjamin kept spreading both legs out, stopping himself along the edges. He gave me a quizzical look and didn't seem too interested in what we were doing. After a few more failed attempts I decided that slides would have to wait.

By now the woman had moved over to the baby swings with her little guy. I decided to head that direction as well, thinking a swing might be something my son would enjoy. The other little boy was already swinging high and giggling in excitement as I got Benjamin settled into his swing. Instead of swinging him high, I kept a hold of the chain handles and gently pushed him back and forth. I had to keep an eye on his mouth to make sure he wasn't sucking on the metal handles. Benjamin seemed to be surprised by this new experience, but he enjoyed watching the other child swing and laugh. At one point I asked the other lady how old the boy was and she said he was three. She asked Benjamin's age, and I told her 21 months. I then commented, "This is his first time to swing. He's still trying to decide what he thinks of it." I wrestled with feelings of self-consciousness, knowing my statement was probably surprising. A moment later I decided to actually let go of the swing handles and just gently push Benjamin. He seemed to do okay, until I glanced away for a moment at some girls who had just run up. In that split second he tried to launch himself to get to me. Thankfully, the swing seat was high enough around him that it held him in place, but images of him tumbling head first onto the ground still crowded into my mind. I decided that was enough swinging for the day and pulled him out.

In one last playground attempt, we headed for the "big kid" swings where I sat down with Benjamin on my lap and slowly rocked. We only lasted a few moments; the swing was uncomfortable and a group of girls were on their way over to play, so I wanted to make room for them. I placed Benjamin back in his stroller and headed for the car. I felt a mixture of emotions. It was wonderful to have some time outside with my son, and I enjoy trying new things with him. However, it was difficult to be reminded of his present delays and the limitations they create. I so look forward to the day when Benjamin can hold my hand as we walk through the park. I look forward to watching him climb and slide and swing. I imagine the smiles and laughter that will accompany these future outings. I know they will come; it just won't be within the time table I once envisioned. As I lifted Benjamin out of his stroller and got ready to place him in his car seat, he smiled and me and squealed. He was so content--so happy to be outside and just spend time with

Mommy. I found myself saying, "Did you have a good time? That's what's important." And it is.

Lessons from a Sippy Cup

"Benjamin, do you want a drink from your cup?" I make the sign for "drink" and "cup" as I pull out his sippy cup full of cold water, slightly sweetened with juice. From his high chair, Benjamin throws up his hands in eager anticipation. As I bring the cup to his mouth, he opens wide and THEN... chews on the spout. A small bit of fluid pours into his mouth, and the majority of it slides right back out, down his chin and into the pocket on his bib. We try again and again and again as we have been trying for the last 4 ½ months. I've heard it said that the definition of insanity is to try the same thing over and over expecting different results. But I'm being too harsh; we have tried many variations all with the same result—a wet baby, a wet bib, and possibly a small amount of swallowing. We have tried multiple cups of different shapes and sizes: hard spouts without the stopper in, fast flows and slow flows, with handles and with no handles, soft spouts that require some work to pull the liquid out, open cups, and straws filled with small amounts of fluid released directly into his mouth. We've even tried going back to bottles, which he rejected before his first birthday and rejects still.

Benjamin sees the cup as a fun game, but if he's thirsty, there's only one acceptable thirst-quencher, and her name is Mommy. Now, don't get me wrong, I love to nurse my son. However, at seventeen months, he is 24 ½ pounds and the size of most two-year-olds, so I desperately want him to be able to receive fluid from a source other than me. Some days, after another seemingly unsuccessful session with the cup I wish I could have my own two-year-old temper tantrum. Visions of throwing the cup across the room and sitting on the floor for a good long cry flood my mind. Then I know it's time to move on to another activity. "I love you, Benjamin," I say as I kiss his face and pull him out of the high chair. We'll try again later.

I know I shouldn't compare, but at times I find myself doing that anyway. I marvel as I watch other children my son's age and younger as they toddle around, grab their cup, take a good long drink, set it down, and continue in their play. I'm amazed at the ease with which they have mastered so many skills, which appear to me at times as nearly insurmountable mountains blocking my son from a "normal" life. At times it's hard not to feel a sting of inferiority, and I wonder, "As they all grow up, how will they treat my son? What will they be doing that he can't do?"

******

. . . Fast forward eight months. . . The day in October 2010 when I began writing this piece, I was seeking a release for the swirling emotions pent up inside me. I intended to bring things back around to a positive note. I was going to write about God's patience with me when I take so long in learning a lesson He's teaching me. I was going to write about His unending love for me in my weakness. I was going to write about His confidence and peace in getting me to where He wants me to be, as opposed to my distressing emotions concerning my son's delays. I never got that far. Around the time I wrote the last question, "What will they be doing that he can't do?" Shawn walked in the room. At this point I had slipped quite deeply into the mire of grief and self-pity. He wisely recommended that I take a break from writing and come back later. Well, I never expected "later" to mean a lapse of eight months, but here we go. . . .

There were many more difficult days as we continued our attempts with the cup. There were the disheartening but truthful comments from the speech therapist that, while Benjamin does make progress, it happens to be slower than the majority of children she's worked with. There were the swinging emotions of enjoying the continued bond of breastfeeding with my son to resentment that I still "had" to nurse as opposed to "choosing" to nurse. There was the physical fatigue of producing so much milk for such a big boy. There was, and some days continues to be, the struggle with comparing Benjamin's development to "typically" developing children. One day, however, we finally received the breakthrough we were praying for.

It was some time after the New Year, but I unfortunately neglected to record the exact month and date. I was sick in bed, and Shawn was giving Benjamin his breakfast in the kitchen. I suddenly heard Shawn exclaim, "Thank You, Jesus! Good job, Benjamin! Daddy's so proud of you!" My heart leaped within me, and I could hardly wait for Shawn to share his news. A few minutes later he came into the bedroom beaming as he excitedly told me that Benjamin had just drank over half his cup! He was actually swallowing the fluid! If I hadn't been sick, I would have probably danced!

Now Benjamin still wasn't (and still isn't) latching on to the spout of his cup and sucking the fluid out. He continues to chew the spout but has learned to retain the fluid. By sometime in March we were able to cut down to three nursing sessions a day, and by May it was down to two. He's still very insistent on nursing first thing in the morning and right before bed. However, at this point I can choose to continue nursing, or I can choose to wean. He is receiving adequate fluid from his cup. There's a big difference emotionally between *choosing* to do something and *having* to do something. Right now I'm just taking things one day at a time.

There have been other challenges and breakthroughs in the sippy cup saga. Once it was apparent that Benjamin was adequately swallowing fluids, our speech therapist had us start working to assist him with holding the cup. We would support him at his elbows so that his hands had to do most of the work. She recommended insisting that he either have assistance in holding his cup or assistance in signing "drink" before we would give it to him. This new endeavor created challenges and humor in itself.

Unfortunately, Benjamin has never been very keen on having to work at things; he prefers that others do the work for him, though that is beginning to change little by little. When he came to the realization that he could get out of having to hold his cup if Mommy helped him sign "drink," he began reaching for my hand after each swallow, so that I could assist him in the sign. It did not occur to him to try to make the sign by himself, though admittedly it would probably have been less work! I was encouraged that he at least understood the concept! I finally had to start hiding my hands under the high chair tray so he would have to reach for his cup. He would hold it by himself for a second or two before it would come crashing down on the tray unless Mommy was supporting his elbows.

Then one day in May, we received another breakthrough. Benjamin held his cup, lowered it, and brought it back up to his mouth. He continued to repeat the process. He was drinking independently!

Some days I still marvel that I can set Benjamin's cup in front of him and clean up in the kitchen while he contentedly drinks his fill. The mountain that felt insurmountable has finally been scaled! There have been some things to learn through the process. Benjamin has had to learn that he cannot throw his cup on the floor when it contains something other than milk. This has been a tearful process; his little heart breaks when Mommy flicks him on the cheek and tells him "no" (which in turn breaks Mommy's heart). Thankfully, though, the discipline is starting to pay off. I have had to learn that I shouldn't let him drink a full cup of milk in one sitting (which he would happily do), if I don't want to see it come back up later. I have learned that diluted juice offered at lunch time only disappears a little, but at supper time it all goes down. Most importantly, I have learned that the greater and longer the struggle, the deeper and happier the celebration!

I am very proud of my son. He has to work so hard to accomplish simple tasks that most of us take for granted. The "natural" stages of development do not come naturally for him; he has to fight for each new milestone. It is very bittersweet knowing that he will face many more challenges and victories as he grows. We just had another recent victory last week when Benjamin started pushing himself up into a sitting position. (It's June 2011 as I write this.) When he was finally able to remain sitting up on his own at fourteen months, I never imagined that it wouldn't be until after his second birthday that he would be able to get himself into that position by himself. I never imagined that I would have a two year old who isn't crawling or saying any words. However, I cannot even begin to describe the pride and the love that swells in my heart as I watch him push up on his little arms with all his might, leg up in the air and finally stabilize himself in an upright position. It has been reason for much celebration in our home!

One of the greatest lessons God is teaching me through my son is to celebrate and cherish the little things. He's teaching me to focus on what He *is* doing, not on what He's *not* doing. He's teaching me to live more in the present. I'm far from mastering these lessons, but thankfully I have a very patient Teacher who knows exactly how to help me develop and grow. I'm even more thankful that He never compares me to others but simply loves and celebrates me every step of the way. His love is perfect; mine is not, but my prayer is that I would reflect His love to Benjamin and to others more and more in the days and years to come.

To Wean or Not to Wean?

It really was a big question. By the time we reached Benjamin's second birthday, this question was beginning to surface more and more now that weaning was actually an option. I loved nursing, but the desire for a second child was growing in me. I knew that I would probably be more likely to conceive once Benjamin was weaned and my hormones had the opportunity to re-align themselves again. His two nursing sessions were more for comfort than anything, but it was still a difficult decision to make. The bond I had with Benjamin through breastfeeding was so precious, especially considering how hard I had to fight to be able to nurture him in this way. It wasn't something I wanted to relinquish until I felt sure of my decision, knowing that once I did it would be final.

Benjamin's birthday was at the end of May, and we continued with our twice daily nursing sessions through the whole month of June. A little way into July, I decided I was ready to complete the weaning process. I thought the easiest session to cut first would be the evening one. So one night, instead of nursing my son, I offered him a cup of milk in his highchair before bed. Shawn and I wondered if he would be fussy when we put him down that night, but to our surprise and relief, he slept all the way through until morning. We continued the morning nursing session for a few more days, but at this point I knew he wasn't getting much milk from me anyway. On July 15, 2011, I decided to take the final step. Shawn got Benjamin up that morning, but instead of bringing him to me in the living room, he took our little boy straight to his highchair where I was waiting with a cup of milk. At first he cried and didn't want it, so we offered him some cereal, which he happily gobbled up, and afterward he contentedly drank his milk. I was surprised at the ease of this transition! It was clear that Benjamin was ready to wean, and though I experienced some sadness, I was ready too. I wrote in my journal the next day,

"Benjamin was officially weaned yesterday. It was and is a bittersweet relief."

In the days and weeks that followed, I experienced some different emotions, but I always felt peace about my decision. Still, I missed the cuddle time that nursing had offered. For most of our nursing relationship, Benjamin cuddled with me even after he was finished drinking. I would make faces and give him kisses, and he would squeal with delight. However, a couple months before I weaned him, this routine was already shifting. As soon as my son was done, he was *done*, and he would begin pushing against me in his attempt to get down to the floor where his toys were. Benjamin was starting to gain a greater measure of independence, and he needed to. In fact, only *three days* after he was weaned, he started his own little version of an army crawl (more on that later)! My boy was quickly leaving his baby days behind him and venturing into the world of toddlerhood! I was relieved by the greater measure of freedom I had as well. If Shawn and I wanted to leave Benjamin with a babysitter while we went out on a date, we didn't have to be back at a certain time for our son to nurse. We could simply leave a cup of milk for him, and he was happy, at least most of the time!

Benjamin continues to gain more independence in his behavior and personality. He is very much a little boy, and he is so much fun! He is still a "Mama's boy," much to Daddy's disappointment, but he is becoming more and more his own little person. I have to take advantage of any cuddle time I can get now, usually when he's sleepy, because he is a little ball of energy, wanting to play and explore. I'm so proud of him! He still enjoys his milk in the morning and the evening, though we have since smoothly transitioned from cow's milk to soy milk, a change that has done wonders for his digestive system.

I look back with gratitude and affection for the two years of breastfeeding I enjoyed with my son and the good nutritional start I was able to give him. I look forward with excitement and pride at the little boy he's growing up to be. And, to be perfectly honest, I look forward with eager anticipation to building that special nursing bond with our next baby, whenever he or she graces our lives in the future.

Defining "Normal"

Shawn calls him "Astro Boy" when he's all strapped in. At first sight I thought it resembled a strange torture device. Benjamin knows it as his movie time place. I know it as his "Super Stand." At this present time, our family knows it as "normal."

When Benjamin's child development specialist first recommended a Super Stand sometime before his first birthday, I couldn't quite envision what she was referring to. She explained that it was very important for Benjamin to have a way to be held in an upright position in order to develop proper posture for future standing and walking and to give him the opportunity to bear down with weight on his feet and legs. Though he was a big boy overall, his feet seemed to be lagging behind. She explained that the body needs weight on the feet to send the message to the bones to grow. Otherwise, the human body will actually take calcium from the bones that are not being used much and send it to other parts of the body. She also said that it's important for his digestive system that he be placed in an upright position more and more, especially since our son has a bad tendency of spitting up. So, she helped us make the proper connections, had measurements taken for Benjamin's equipment, and filled out the necessary paperwork to make a requisition to our insurance company. Thankfully we were approved, though it was several months before his Super Stand actually arrived.

By this time we had just recently moved into our newly purchased home. Benjamin had just learned to remain in a sitting position by himself. He had already received ankle braces (known as orthotics) for use throughout the day but most importantly for when he would be in his stander. The importance of his orthotics did not sink in for me, however, for several more months. They left red marks on his feet and ankles, and he seemed so uncomfortable that I did not have a very strong resolve to make him use them much. By the time I realized how important they are for Benjamin to develop proper foot alignment and ankle strength that will set a life-long course for his posture and walking stance, it was time to have new ones made. They only recently came in.

Anyway, back to the stander…A gentleman delivered the large contraption to our home and showed us how to use it. He helped us make the necessary adjustments for Benjamin's current size and taught us how to make future adjustments. I probably looked like I was a deer trapped in headlights as he told us more than once, "I know it looks intimidating, but it's really quite simple." "Simple" was the last word in my mind at that moment! How simple would it be to strap my 15-month-old into this device every day and listen to him scream? We were encouraged to start Benjamin out in small increments with the goal of increasing his time to at least an hour a day, though it didn't have to be all at once. Knowing time in the stander would be important for our son's development and thankful that such an expensive piece of equipment had been provided for us, we pressed forward. I have to admit, though, that in some ways this large and awkward piece felt more like an intrusion in both my house and my heart. It was difficult to hear Benjamin's cries of protest and see his tear-streaked face as we tried to familiarize him with this brand new experience that must become a part of our "normal" life. It was painful that he would even need such a seemingly drastic intervention when other children his age were up and running around. After some rocky first attempts, though, we discovered that our son seemed to forget, at least in part, about the awkwardness of the stander when we played one of his favorite baby movies. Soon his cries of protest evolved into occasional cries of impatience while I strapped him in, so eager he was to watch Vinko the Bear and D.J. the Dinosaur from *Baby Geniuses*, and later Rachel from *Baby Signing Time*, Elmo from *Sesame Street*, or Ta, Dee and Ed from *Musical Baby*.

What felt so intrusive and so foreign has now become a part of our daily routine. Benjamin watches a movie in his stander every morning while Mommy gets cleaned up, and he watches another one or two throughout the afternoon and early evening. Overall, he averages around two hours of stander time every day. Instead of tears, I see smiles as I push the hydraulic lever to raise him up while telling him, "We're going up, up, up!" or later "Down, down, down." Benjamin has accepted his stander as part of "normal" life and has no concept of how "abnormal" our routine would appear to the general population. While I still have this awareness, the stander is now part of "normal" life for me as well. I've nearly mastered the art of maneuvering the bulky piece from behind his crib's headboard out into the living room and back again, though the patches of chipped paint at the bottom of the doorway reveal my many less successful attempts. Benjamin's orthotic braces are becoming "normal" too. He's not to the point of being able to wear them all day, but he no longer fights me when I put them on his feet, though he doesn't necessarily like having to sit still during the process. During the first drawn-out attempts while he cried and fought and I felt like I was all thumbs, I just kept telling my son (more for myself than anything), "We have to get used to these. It's part of life now, and that's just the way it's going to be." We're beginning to adjust much better, and I can see the improvements the orthotic braces are making in his ability and stamina to remain in an assisted standing position.

These unusual interventions are never what I pictured, and they're not necessarily easy, but that doesn't mean they are not good. I'm realizing more and more that so many of life's disappointments spring from the root of unmet expectations. I have an expectation for what "normal" should look like; when that expectation is not met, it is easy to feel hurt, angry, and/or offended. It's easy to feel like I'm "missing out" on something I feel the "right" to have. However, am I really missing out, or do I just need to alter my expectations? What should my expectations look like anyway? Life is uncertain; God is unchanging. Life (in this age) is fleeting; God is eternal. He is the same yesterday, today and forever (Hebrews 13:8). He has promised to never leave me or forsake me (Hebrews 13:5). He has promised that His love for me is unconditional; nothing can separate me from His love (Romans 8:38-39). He has promised that His goodness and His mercy will pursue me and overtake me if I will allow Him access to my heart (Psalm 23:6). Maybe my expectation should be to love Him and trust in His love for me no matter what I'm faced with in my circumstances (Proverbs 3:5). Maybe my expectation should be in His goodness and eternal wisdom that I most certainly will never fully understand in this life (Isaiah 55:9). Maybe my expectation should be in the glories of the age to come and not in the sufferings of the present age (2 Corinthians 4:18). I say "maybe," but I know it's true.

But now, O Lord, You are our Father; We are the clay, and Your our potter; And all we are the work of Your hand, (Isaiah 64:8). He has us all in a process, and each one's process looks different. Some steps are delightful, and some steps are painful. Will we yield ourselves to His process, or will we insist on our own way and grow hardened if we do not receive it? Will we allow the disappointments of our unmet expectations in life beat us down or will we allow Him to use these things to shape and mold our hearts as He sees fit? One of my greatest prayers is that my heart would stay tender in Jesus' hands. What He wants is the inner response of my heart towards Him in trust and love no matter the circumstances. This is the only thing that will truly give me the strength to stand.

Embracing Change

The Holy Spirit often speaks to me through my son. This morning I heard His voice again. Every morning while I shower and get ready for the day, Benjamin watches a movie in his Super Stand. Most mornings I pop in one of his two Sesame Street DVDs. Yesterday, while running an errand I happened upon a brand new baby DVD. It appeared to be the same genre as some of Benjamin's other movies, with lots of music, puppets, and images of infants and children playing. I thought it would be very nice to have another option for his viewing enjoyment (and for Mommy's sanity!), so I made the purchase. Shortly after we arrived at home, I set Benjamin up in his stander and popped in his new movie, while I got busy preparing supper. Now, my son is very much a creature of habit. He most often bucks against any new thing at the start. However, with persistence, he will eventually embrace the change and keep moving forward. (Do you hear the lesson yet?) So, I expected some protest to the new movie, and it surely happened. He did the same thing with his now beloved Sesame Street shows, among others. The fine line for me is being able to recognize how much he can handle at once, and I am still very much in the process of learning! So, after 10 minutes of hearing his cries of protest, I stopped the movie and popped in one of his favorites instead. After that, he was as happy as a clam. I told him, "We'll try it again tomorrow." Well, back to this morning—we gave his new movie another chance while I got ready for the day. I could hear his disgruntled cries even in the shower. By the time I was dressed, Holy Spirit was already speaking to me as my son was escalating in his discontent. We made it through over 20 minutes this morning, and I am confident that in time this new DVD will encourage smiles instead of cries.

As I listened to my child, I felt like the Lord was whispering to me about how often His children (myself included) do the same thing when He ushers change into our lives. It's so easy to remain in our comfort zones with what's familiar. However, we will never move forward with God if we stay in that place. Sometimes the changes are circumstantial and out of our control. We can gripe and complain and fall into self-pity, or we can fix our eyes on Jesus, place our trust in Him, and keep moving forward. Sometimes the changes are optional—a new attitude of heart, a willingness to embrace a new mindset, or a willingness to go in the direction we feel He's asking us to go, even when it means giving up our own agendas. Change is often hard, and it's often uncomfortable, but He always has our best interest at heart. However, if we buck and protest, He will allow us to stay where we are for a season. He will not cross our free will. He will be persistent, though, and bring us back to the place of choice again and again, not content to leave us where we are. His leadership over our lives is perfect, but we have to be willing to relinquish control. If I'm not confident in His heart of love towards me, this is a very scary thing. The more I experience His love and His affections towards me, the easier it becomes to trust and allow Him to lead. In fact, refusing to allow Him to have His way becomes a scarier prospect than losing my control! Only He sees from eternity past to eternity future, and only He loves with perfection.

There was another lesson to be learned through my son this morning. His cries of anger and frustration effectively *pushed out* quite a mess! I smelled it as soon as I started to lower him down in his stander. Now, this may be more information than you care to know, but when I say mess I mean MESS! We are talking about the kind of blow-out that necessitated an immediate bath, load of laundry and sanitation of his changing pad. It's a wonder I made it through the incident without needing a fresh change of clothes myself! Again I heard the Holy Spirit's gentle voice. *I love you and enjoy you even when you're making messes.* Oh, He's good! Often the process of change brings the messes up and out. Things I didn't even realize were in my heart begin to surface, and it stinks! It's so easy at this point to slip into feelings of shame and condemnation, but Jesus already bore all my shame on the cross. He is not intimidated by my messes, and I believe He thoroughly enjoys the process of cleaning me up because He knows exactly where He's taking me, and He sees me through His blood that has already washed me clean and pure. There is a processing of "working out my salvation" (Philippians 2:12-13), but He sees ahead into eternity future when I will be fully conformed to His image, and He enjoys me in the here and now.

I suppose this is where my analogy breaks down a bit. I cannot say that there was any enjoyment for me in cleaning up my son's stinky mess. I didn't enjoy the process, but I most definitely enjoy the child!

Water Baby

Benjamin is a water baby. He loves to be wet! Bath times have almost always been an enjoyable experience. He loves to watch the water running out of the faucet. He loves to see the light reflecting in the water, and he gets his face down so close, studying the surface from all different angles. He loves to splash. He loves to have me pour water over him, especially on his hands and feet. Rubber duckies make the experience even more exciting. At the end of bath time, he's fascinated by the water going down the drain and has even started sliding onto his belly to get a closer look.

Recently Benjamin had his first pool therapy session with his new physical therapist Rebecca. I think it is safe to say it was the most enjoyable therapy session of his life thus far (and he's had plenty). He smiled and squealed and didn't even mind getting his face in the water a bit. Rebecca encouraged me to give him lots of opportunities to be in the water. I knew she was planning a swim night for her client families at the local mini water park/pool, and I was sure to mark the calendar so we could be there tonight. As it turned out, Shawn had an end of the summer event tonight for his summer day camp program. His event began at 6:00, and the pool party began at 7:00. I attended his program until the reception, and then headed with Benjamin to the pool, where Shawn would later meet us.

Benjamin thought we'd walked into a dream land! There was a kiddie pool that led into a larger pool, (no deep end), and there was so much to see and experience: cascading water, mini water spouts, slides, etc. He demonstrated his delight unhindered for an entire hour before his daddy was even able to arrive. We sat in the water, played with the water spouts, floated around the baby pool in a baby floating device and chatted with other families. If Benjamin could speak, I think he would have exclaimed, "Mommy, why didn't we come here sooner? Can we do this every day?!"

When Shawn arrived we were walking around in the big pool. He got changed and happily joined us, then took Benjamin around the whirl pool (a circular canal with a gentle current that helps push you along). We placed him in a flotation device again and walked him all over the place. We had a wonderful time as a family, and it was such a delight to see Benjamin so obviously enjoying himself until he was just too tired to know what to do anymore. (The pool party surpassed his normal bedtime!) It was also special to see so many other families with their children of all different ages and ability levels enjoying some quality time together: a tiny baby who is six months old but born four months premature, a young man who was being walked around in the pool by his mother, some children who had no apparent disabilities, children with Down syndrome and spinal bifida, and older children/teens who appeared to need complete assistance in every area of functioning.

I realized again tonight that we have so much to be thankful for. I want to spend much more time rejoicing in Benjamin's abilities than in grieving his delays. I don't want to take for granted his smiles and squeals and contagious little personality. I also want to learn to see all people through God's eyes, regardless of their outward appearance. The Lord was speaking to me about this earlier in the week. When I look at Benjamin, though I'm aware of his disabilities, I don't see a disability; I see my son whom I love so intensely. I can't help but love him because he came from me, and he's mine. I felt the Father whisper, "You may look at someone and see their areas of bondage and sin; I look at them and see the child I so dearly love. They came from My very heart. I can't help Myself but to love them!" God isn't focused on *our disabilities* but on *His ability* to transform us with His love. Whether the disability is internal or external, I want to see the beauty of each life from Heaven's eyes. I welcome Him to bring more of these "water lessons" my way!

The Power of Weakness

Author's Note: In the summer of 2011, Shawn and I came to the end of our season at The Salvation Army, and with the blessing and support of our pastors there we stepped into the next thing God had in store for us. The Night Watch prayer gathering we had been a part of for several years birthed a new church in town called the International House of Prayer-Bartlesville (IHOP-B), and we were asked to join the leadership team. The references to our church from here on speak of IHOP-B.

In many ways, I feel as though in the last two and a half years I have been in a school of weakness, yet sometimes I think I may still be in kindergarten. Becoming a new parent and raising a child with special needs has caused me to recognize my own weaknesses and limitations in ways potentially nothing else could have done. Observing the weaknesses in my young son over the months and now years has taught me more about the kindness of God and His unconditional love for weak human beings. The lessons, though still elementary, have been invaluable.

I have so many thoughts spinning right now with what direction I should take in writing, so I guess I will go with what's been right in front of me. This last month especially I feel like God has been highlighting weakness to me on so many levels. He is inviting me to embrace my weakness without shame and to completely rely on His love and strength. Near the end of September our church embarked on a 21 day Daniel fast (no meats, sweets, or choice foods), and a handful of us met nightly to pray and seek the Lord. We were fasting to see breakthrough on many levels: in our personal lives, in our church, in our city, in our nation, and even around the globe. As we came together night after night feeling more physically and emotionally weak from the fasting, one thing became undeniably clear—we have NOTHING apart from Jesus

Our need of Him is so deep, so far reaching into every sphere and pocket of life. There is nothing we have to bring to Him that He didn't first give to us, including our love for Him (see 1 John 4:19).

My physical sense of weakness was increasingly heightened before, during, and even now after the fast. Days before the beginning of our fast, I had an unexpected recurrence of what I thought was severe acid reflux. Over the next few weeks I had a handful of episodes that left me screaming in pain on the floor, in addition to daily feeling at least some level of discomfort every time I ate. Near the end of the fast I discovered through a series of events, including an ER visit, that I had been misdiagnosed for the last two years. While I had been treating myself for acid reflux, my gallbladder was filling up with more and more stones, to the point that almost anything could trigger an attack. I consulted with a surgeon, and a week after completing our fast I went in for outpatient laparoscopic surgery to have my gallbladder removed. That was four days ago, and I am still very weak physically. Shawn has been caring for me and Benjamin, as I am not able to pick up our son yet. My mom is on an airplane as I write this to come help me for the week since Shawn has to return to work. Friends have offered prayers, encouragement, and food while I recover. The physical limitations and discomfort have been frustrating, but again I am faced with my own weakness and my need for Jesus and for the Body of Christ.

I have been realizing more and more how quickly I try to rely on my own strength and ability, my own understanding of things, and my own emotions and opinions, which can so easily be swayed. Physical wellness impacts emotional wellness, and both can fluctuate so quickly. I am becoming more and more convinced that I can't rely on what I *feel* but only on what God's Word *says*, for His Word is unchanging. Yet, I so often look to myself or others when faced with a need instead of acknowledging my complete barrenness apart from Jesus. He wants me to come to Him in my weakness and vulnerability, to throw myself on His mercy and grace and all-sufficiency. How easily I forget that He loves weak, powerless human beings, and He rises to show Himself strong on our behalf. Indeed, it is in the very acknowledgment of my complete lack that He steps in with His complete abundance. All He wants is that I trust Him absolutely, yielding myself to His ways that are always superior to my own.

I learn so much watching Benjamin. He doesn't worry or fear but has a simple trust that Mommy and Daddy are going to take care of him. He doesn't consider his inabilities to meet his own needs and try to plot how to get around them. He doesn't question where his provision is coming from or try to figure things out before they happen. He lives in the present moment, confident that he is loved and cared for, free to be himself and to learn and grow. He demonstrates to me day in and day out the simplicity of a child's trust. I was recently reading in a book called *The Seeking Heart* by the 17th century Fenelon and was struck by the following:

"Your only task is to bear the weakness of your body and mind. Strength is made perfect in weakness. You are only strong in God when you are weak in yourself. Your weakness will be your strength if you accept it with a lowly heart...

Trusting in God is a simple resting in God's love, as a baby lies in its mother's arms...

The point of trusting God is not to do great things that you can feel good about, but to trust God from a place of deep weakness. Here is a way to know if you've actually trusted God with something—you will not think about the matter any longer, nor will you feel a lack of peace."

Like the apostle Paul, I want to know in reality, not just in theory, that His power truly is made perfect in my weakness (2 Cor. 12:9). The all-powerful, eternal God promises to dwell with those who are contrite and lowly of heart, recognizing their absolute need of Him (Isaiah 57:15). I want to live close to His heart. It's time to know and embrace the power of weakness!

Work Cited

Fenelon. *The Seeking Heart.* Jacksonville, FL: SeedSowers Publishing. Print. Vol. 4 of *Library of Spiritual Classics.* 66.

Someday

Someday Benjamin will learn to stand. Someday he will be able to walk next to me, holding my hand instead of being carried everywhere. Someday he will be able to run to his daddy when he comes home from work. Someday he will be able to say "Mommy" and "Daddy"; he will be able to articulate words and form sentences to communicate his thoughts and feelings. Someday he will be able to feed himself without assistance. Someday he will no longer need diapers. Someday he will have developed the necessary motor skills to throw and catch a ball, to go down a slide, to ride a tricycle, to color a picture, to make a simple craft, etc. Some days the longing for "someday" is more deeply felt than others. Today has been one of those days…

This morning we had an appointment at the local health department with Benjamin's audiologist to have casts made for new ear molds for his hearing aids. This is never a pleasant process. I have to hold his arms down and keep his head as still as possible while she examines his ears one at a time. After examining each ear, she pushes a small piece of cotton with a string attached to it down deep into the ear canal in order to protect his inner ear. She then fills the ear with soft putty that looks remarkably like Laffy Taffy, though I'm sure it doesn't taste the same! This has to stay in place for a few minutes while it hardens to create a cast of Benjamin's ear. The casts are then sent in to a lab that will make his new molds, which we will hopefully be able to pick up in a few weeks. My son hates this process. He doesn't like things in his ears (other than his hearing aids, and on some days he doesn't like them), and he struggles the whole time. Being held down makes him angry, so by the time the whole process was complete this morning, he was a mess of tears and snot. I was hopeful that our next activity would be a welcome distraction that would cheer him up.

The local health department hosts monthly play groups, each highlighting a different theme. Today was the Christmas play group, with multiple crafts, snacks, and a free book from Santa Claus. I had been planning for a few weeks to take Benjamin with the hope that he would enjoy being around other children and be able to gain some new experiences. The audiologist walked us down the hall to the center of the activity. My son was still teary-eyed, and the commotion of the busy play group seemed to only add to his distress instead of capturing his interest. As I carried him around, examining the different craft options, he continued to fuss and cry, and I felt like all eyes were on me (though that may have just been in my head more than anything). All of the tables were being manned by students from the local technical college.

I decided to start at a table that was set up to make pasta necklaces, with dry noodles painted red and green. I awkwardly held Benjamin, trying to talk to him about the craft as I slid noodles over a covered wire. I finished it quickly, and the students helped to secure it around my son's neck. He was not impressed. Within 5-10 minutes he managed to rip it off, scattering noodles on the floor. Some of the pieces were broken in the process, and his necklace found its final destination in the trash can. Sigh…

After making the necklace, we headed over to a play corner that was really designed for babies, but I hoped a musical toy would calm him down and hopefully alter his crabby mood. It was not to be. Benjamin pushed away the toy I tried to entice him with and continued to cry, while a baby about a third of his size sat and played contentedly. I started lifting him up over my head and kissing his tummy which scored me some smiles and giggles, but it was short lived. As soon as our little game was over, the fussing resumed.

We made our way to another table set up to make candy canes with pipe cleaners and red and white beads. We didn't even begin this craft. Benjamin tried to dump all the beads on the floor, but we caught him in time, and he continued to throw his fit. I awkwardly excused us and headed to the side of the room to chat with a few of the coordinators, explaining the effects of his audiologist appointment. It was during this time that the pasta necklace met its demise. They understood, and I knew I didn't have to justify my son's behavior, but I was feeling both disappointed and embarrassed.

My next idea was a trip to the bathroom to give him a brief change of scenery. This appeared to work, until we re-emerged into the play group room and Benjamin began to cry *again*. Now, at this point I should have gotten us bundled up and headed home. I had really been looking forward to this morning, though, so I held on to the hope that something would capture his attention, and we could make a fun memory together. I decided to sit down with him for a few minutes so he could just observe things from a safe place and chatted with the woman beside me. I was waiting for a spot to open at a craft table where we could make an ornament and a Christmas door hanger using foam stickers. When a chair opened up, we headed that way. I was hoping Benjamin would enjoy placing the stickers, but he had no interest and continued to fuss while I quickly made him an ornament and a door hanger and tried to talk to him about it step by step.

At this point I knew there really was no use in staying. I did want to get him a free book from Santa, so while we waited for one child to finish his turn, I took my son to a station where a young woman was hot-gluing pom-poms onto Popsicle stick snowflakes to make Christmas ornaments. Each child could pick out the colors they wanted. Benjamin was slightly interested in pulling handfuls of pom-poms out of the bags, but his idea was to then throw them on the floor. He had tried to throw multiple things on the floor by this point and had succeeded with some, including the door hanger

Mommy was working on and his right hearing aid. The young woman quickly finished his ornament and handed it to me. I was happy that Benjamin at least played a part in picking out the colors, even if it was by default.

We headed over to Santa's corner, and his "elf" presented my son with a small book. He asked us a bit about our Christmas plans and tried to get Benjamin to give him a high-five. My son just looked at him not knowing what to think and continued his complaints. I knew I had kept us there way too long. We got our coats on, I strapped Benjamin in his stroller, and we made our way for the door. As we crossed the room, I looked longingly at all the small children happily making crafts and walking from table to table. I knew many of them were probably close to my son's age, some older, some younger. I felt so alone. "Well, we tried," I said to one of the coordinators as we reached the doors. She encouraged me "That's all you can do," and gave me a flyer listing dates and themes for future play groups. I thanked her and we went on our way.

I felt such disappointment in my heart as we drove home. I recognized some of my own selfishness too. Did I want the experience for my son's benefit or for my own? When he didn't respond in the way I wanted him to, I was upset. He hasn't reached the "somedays" I dream about yet, and I can't make him get there on my timetable. Today I've been reminding myself that while it's okay to look forward to the somedays, I don't want that longing to rob me of the ability to enjoy my todays. I want to cherish every season of my son's life, knowing that there will be joys and frustrations, victories and obstacles all along the way. The somedays I dream about now will eventually be only distant memories, and new somedays will appear on the horizon. There is treasure to be found in today, though, and wisdom to be gleaned if I maintain a teachable heart. All of my todays and all of my somedays are given as a gift to prepare me for the great Someday, when my faith will truly be made sight, and I see my Jesus face to face. I want to live in anticipation of that Someday, and I want to raise my son to do the same. His disability is but for a moment; his wholeness will be for eternity.

The Comparison Game

In the comparison game, no one ever really wins. If I come out feeling *better than*, it only feeds an unhealthy pride. If I come out feeling *less than*, discouragement and self-pity are right around the corner. Either outcome brings greater bondage, not greater freedom. Neither outcome brings me closer to the heart of Jesus. Knowing this first-hand, why am I so quick to slip into this deadly game again and again? This morning I found myself in the familiar struggle…

Shawn and I have been trying (unsuccessfully so far) to conceive a second child for a year's time now. We tried two years for Benjamin. The disappointments of those two years were very painful. The disappointments of this last year have been as well. Then, a few days ago I had an unexpected and frightening attack of the same nature as the gall bladder attacks I was suffering from prior to my surgery last October. I didn't think that was even possible, but there I was getting sick in the bathroom and screaming in agonizing pain on the floor while Shawn raced to get Benjamin ready so he could drive me to the ER. It also happened to be the day that my menstrual cycle was scheduled to start, so before I could be treated, the lab had to run a pregnancy test. I wrestled back and forth with my emotions as we waited for the results. I so long to be pregnant again, but I also wanted to be able to take some pain medicine and have the CT scan run on my stomach to find out what in the world was going on with my body. The pregnancy test results were negative, and the medical staff continued treating me. The CT scan revealed no problems with my appendix (one of the initial fears) and no evidence of stones in the duct connecting my liver to my intestine. The ER doctor concluded that I must have a build-up of "sludge" (a highly medical term, I know, that refers to the presence of microscopic stones) in the duct from my liver to my intestines. So, I was instructed to continue a low-fat diet, take the pain medicine left over from my surgery as necessary, and call my surgeon on Monday (tomorrow). He can look at the results of my CT scan and decide what steps need to be taken next. Sigh...

This morning the disappointment of another false pregnancy test, coupled with the unexpected medical complications was really weighing on my heart. Before I knew it, I was playing the comparison game. Why do so many women, who may not even be trying to get pregnant, conceive so easily while we continue to try month after month? Why do so many women give birth to healthy baby after healthy baby when our son has had so many medical problems? Why am I fast approaching my 30th birthday with only one child when there are so many women younger than me who already have multiple children? Why am I having the medical complications I do when I'm living a healthier lifestyle than many of the people around me? It appears to be only another road block in my desire to conceive. What about the countless unborn lives that are murdered daily in the name of "convenience" and "freedom of choice?" I so want to bring a new life into the world and cherish that life as a precious treasure from God. I also long for the experience of raising a "typically developing" child who will naturally achieve new milestones without the intensity of intervention, work, and tears that we experience with Benjamin. What would it feel like to bring home a healthy baby after a safe delivery? Why is that the expected norm for so many and still only a distant dream for me? Pretty soon I was in an emotional tailspin. I knew where I was going and that it wasn't helping me at all, but it was a struggle to come up and out.

During our worship at church this morning we sang about the cross of Jesus Christ and the immense love He demonstrated to us. As I sang and played my guitar, I pictured Jesus' passion in my mind's eye and thought, "How can the One who poured out His life blood in love for me, not be trusted with every aspect of my heart and life?" I reminded myself of something He gently spoke to my heart a few months ago, as I poured out my longing to Him for a second child:

Do not waste this time but fill your heart with the oil of intimacy. Cherish this time and be content in Me. It is My gift to you.

I know that when our second child comes, the busyness and demands on my time will significantly increase. I know that the one-on-one attention I've been able to give Benjamin has been so valuable, especially in light of his many delays. I know that the time I've already had to fight for to get alone with Jesus has been a gift. He is inviting me to go deeper into His heart during this season of waiting. Even the uncertainty of my medical condition can be a place to lean into Him more. The comparison game robs me of these truths. In the comparison game the attitude of my heart accuses God, (though I may not say it with my mouth) instead of trusting Him. It lies to me that He is unjust, that He is withholding good from me, and that He doesn't care. I know these things are not true, but how quickly my emotions can be drawn in this direction if I do not take my thoughts captive and bring them back to Jesus.

Life's trials and disappointments can spring from many sources. There is an enemy of our souls who is out to steal, kill and destroy. There are the consequences of our own poor choices or the poor choices of people in our lives. There are the inevitable and natural ups and downs of life that no person is immune to. There is also the loving discipline of the Lord, which He uses to draw our hearts back to Him if we have strayed away or to mature us in our walk with Him. Whatever the source of the suffering, though, Jesus desires to use it all to bring us to a place of greater intimacy with Him. He always has the end in mind; He sees past the temporal and into eternity; surely He can be trusted with every facet of our lives!

Will I recognize the gifts of God in my life when they come packaged in a way I did not expect or request? Will I be thankful for and receive His gifts when they look different from what I wanted? Do I believe that I have a better handle on what my life should look like than my Creator, who knows all and loves me without reservation? Will I still hope in His promises when everything around me seems to be screaming the opposite? Will I genuinely trust the One who left heavenly glory to identify with my own weakness and brokenness and to pour out His life for me that I may be made whole?

I'm so thankful that Jesus is not surprised by my emotional struggles. He is not offended by my weakness when I find myself slipping into the comparison game--again. He is patient and tender towards me in my brokenness, but He is not content to leave me there. He is inviting me to life and freedom, though I must choose to respond. Some scriptures went through my mind this morning as I wrestled through my emotions:

Shall the clay say to him who forms it, 'What are you making?' Or shall the handiwork say, 'He has no hands?' (Isaiah 45:9b).

After the risen Jesus prophesied to Peter about the martyr's death he would face to glorify God, Peter looked at John...

Peter, seeing him, said to Jesus, "But Lord, what about this man?" Jesus said to him, "If I will that he remain till I come, what is that to you? You follow Me," (John 21:21-22).

Lord Jesus, give me grace, whatever my path may look like, to follow closely after You.

The Essence of Benjamin

One of the greatest joys of watching my son grow has been seeing the emergence of his delightful little personality, which has really started to shine! At the time I write this Benjamin is a little over two-and-a-half, and I wonder at how quickly the time has gone by. On the other hand, though, it's so hard to imagine life without him. His exuberant laugh and contagious smile have brightened many a person's day, especially his mommy's! That is not to say that all times are filled with laughs and smiles; he definitely knows how to demonstrate the temper of a two-year-old. Benjamin releases the full expression of whatever emotion he is experiencing at any given time, without reservation or shame. A few pages of writing could never do justice to describing all of my little guy's personhood, but it is my goal to at least capture the *essence* of who Benjamin is during this stage of his life.

I think the best way to accomplish this goal is to describe a typical day in our lives. Any time between 5:00-6:00 am, Benjamin announces to the world that he is awake and ready to begin his day, as evidenced by his cries of protest from his crib. He's awake, so everyone else should be as well, right? Now if it's too close to the 5:00 hour, Mommy and Daddy are content to allow our early riser to fuss/play/hopefully sleep in his crib a while longer. Once the lights are flipped on in his room, the fussing ceases as he turns his head toward the door in anticipation. If he woke up in a good mood, there are smiles and squeals as one of us pulls him out of the crib and proceeds to change his diaper. If he woke up in a bad mood, he continues in his complaint throughout his diaper change as if to say, *"Hurry it up already! I want my breakfast!"*

As we approach his high chair, his little legs are already kicking in anticipation. Most morning meals consist of a sippy cup of soy milk mixed with chocolate or vanilla vitamin powder and a warm bowl of oatmeal with fruit mixed in. As I scoop up each bite of oatmeal, I hand the spoon to Benjamin to feed himself, which he is fully capable of doing. Some days, though, he tries to hide his hands underneath his highchair tray, hoping Mommy won't notice and will do the work for him! "Hold your spoon, Benjamin," I coach. He eventually consents. Most bites of oatmeal (or any food he particularly enjoys) are accompanied by his personal commentary of "Mmmm!"

Once breakfast is over, I clean up his face and tray, brush his teeth (which he usually thinks is funny), and we head into the living room for play time. I already have an array of toys scattered across the floor to encourage him to crawl. I sit on the couch with my coffee, Bible, and journal and try to have some quiet time while Benjamin happily plays. Every few minutes at least he looks at me and grins, wanting to make sure I'm watching him. Music toys and balls are his favorite. He sets off one of his favorite songs and begins to bob his head up and down, dancing to the tune. He loves to dance! Musical toys, Daddy's Scooby Doo cell phone ringtone, and Mommy's guitar quickly incite his animated movement. Sometimes he dances when no music is playing, and I wonder if he is grooving to the tune in his head. Other times he creates his own music for dance, "Aaaa-aa-aa-aa. Aaaa-aa-aa-aa!" He also loves hand clapping and rhythm of any kind. He will often stick his hand in between my own as I clap out a rhythm for him. Maybe he will follow in my footsteps one day and play percussion (one of my biggest passions during my school years).

After awhile, checking in with Mommy from across the room is not enough. Laughing, he makes his way toward the couch and attempts to pull up. With a little bit of assistance he pulls to a stand and squeals with delight as I pick him up to cuddle. One of my first exclamations to follow is usually, "Nice touch, Benjamin!" This is an area we are working on. Benjamin loves faces and hair, and in his enthusiasm, he tends to grab, slap and sometimes claw the face in front of him or pull hair by the handful. He doesn't mean to cause any harm; every ounce of him is expressing his excitement, but the results can be painful. I hold his hand flat and gently stroke it down my cheek while saying, "Nice touch. Nice touch." He smiles and buries his face in my shoulder. I cover him with kisses, and he laughs and squeals. He loves to make a "fake" laugh, "Ah-ah-ah-ah-ah-ah-ah" and get Mommy to mimic him. I say "Give me five!" at which he smiles and slaps my hand. After a few moments of cuddles, he's ready to get back down on the floor and continue to play.

Before long, I see him crawling to the basket of board books at the end of the couch. If I don't notice fast enough, he lays down in front of the basket and begins his "fake" cry, "Ahaa, ahaa, ahaa!" or "Yaaa, yaaa, yaaa!" with right hand fingers in his mouth. "Benjamin, do you want to read books with Mommy?" I ask as I pull him into my lap. He places his hands together, palms up, making the sign for "book." I pull out two at a time and hold them in front of him. "Which one do you want to read?" He pushes the rejected book to the side. Reading is one of my son's favorite activities. He especially loves lift-the-flap and texture books. I have most if not all of them memorized by heart since we have read them so many times. He could read and read and read. When we reach the end of our stack, I must quickly divert his attention to a new activity, or I am met with cries of protest.

When I'm ready to take my shower and get ready for the day, I pull out Benjamin's blue Super Stand. When he sees it, he knows it's time to watch a movie, and he's ready! I fit his feet into his orthotic braces, pull on his shoes, and strap him into the stander. He smiles as I push him up using the hydraulic system and tell him, "We're going up, up, up!" He doesn't like waiting for the movie to start; he thinks it's never fast enough. Once I have one of his favorite shows going, he is content, and I head for the shower. His movies tend to run about thirty minutes each, so I will often pop in a second one, giving me a little more time to finish getting ready and to get some things done around the house. By the end of his second movie, Benjamin is ready for a break from the stander. As I lower him down and unstrap him I ask, "Benjamin do you want to take a bath?" while making the sign for "bath." He smiles, knowing what this means.

As we head down the hall to the bathroom, my little guy is kicking his legs in anticipation again. He loves bath time! I set him on the floor by the tub while I start running the water. His eagerness is building. While I don't particularly like that we have a carpeted bathroom (the house came that way, and we haven't been able to do a remodel yet), I am thankful for it at bath time. Benjamin often wants to hurry me along in the process of getting him in the tub by simply falling backwards, letting me know he is ready for me to take his pajamas off. As soon as his diaper is off, he explodes into laughter as I say "Naked boy!" and set him in the tub. As the tub continues to fill, and I begin to pour water over him, he watches the faucet in fascination, cocking his head from side to side or sliding to his tummy to get a better look. After scrubbing him with baby wash and rinsing him off, it is time to play with the big bath cup I use to rinse him. He loves it when I pour water in front of him. He places one hand and then the other into the flow. We play this game until my arm starts to get tired, and then I pull out the rubber ducks. He has three in particular that are his favorites. I use this opportunity to practice more sign language with him. "Benjamin, are you *playing* with your *ducks* in the *water*? What does the *duck* say? Quack, quack! How many *ducks* do you have? *One, two, three ducks!*" or "Benjamin, are you taking a *bath* in the *water*? Are you *playing* in the *water*? Is it *bath time*? Are you getting *clean* in the *water*?" He absolutely loves it.

When it's time to pull the plug, my little guy slips to his tummy and watches the drain in fascination or continues to play with his ducks until I say "Are you ready to come with *Mommy*?" He reaches for me and laughs again as I transfer him from the tub to his towel and proceed to dry him off. Once a fresh diaper is in place, it's time to put on his lotion. He laughs even more as I sing him the "Lotion Song," set to the tune of one of his favorite *Baby Signing Time* songs. (Oh, the things that you come up with when you're a stay-home mom.)

Lotion, lotion, lotion on my big boy! (I used to sing "baby")

Lotion, lotion, lotion on my big boy!

Lotion, lotion, lotion on my big boy!

Lotion on my big boy!

I put some lotion on Big Boy B, so he will be soft and cuddly

I put some lotion on Big Boy B, and I rub it in his skin after bath time!

I dress him for the day and sit him up to comb his hair, his *least* favorite part. Though Benjamin loves to cuddle, he hates to have his hair messed with. I quickly comb through his hair, holding down his flailing hands and ignoring his grunts of complaint. It's over soon enough, and I pick him up to admire himself in the mirror. "Look! There's Benjamin! He's a clean boy!" He smiles at his reflection, smiles at me, usually grabs my face again, and we head back to the living room.

Soon it's time for a mid-morning snack. Using signs, I ask "Benjamin, are you *hungry*? Do you want to *eat*?" Those words always get his attention! Once settled in his high chair, I place a few handfuls of Multi-grain Cheerios on his tray, and he begins happily munching. He likes to play with them too, sliding his hand back and forth across the tray or kicking the bottom of the tray and watching them bounce. Between his play and messy finger-feeding, my kitchen floor is soon covered with Cheerios, as is my son. In fact, at times I feel my whole house is covered in Cheerios since I'm always finding stray ones in random places throughout the day.

Once snack time is over, it's usually time for a nap. I lay him in his crib with his neon, multi-colored stuffed gorilla (the only stuffed animal he seems to care for at this point), and turn on his little star projector that plays music. On a good day, this is a smooth transition and he happily drifts to sleep--on a *good* day. On some days, Benjamin is convinced a nap is *not* a good idea, and he fusses in his crib until he finally gives in to sleep. There are occasional days, where his will is stronger, and I find him sitting up in his crib an hour later having *never* slept. These are rough days with an inevitable afternoon nap that often has to be cut short to head to a physical therapy appointment or some other unavoidable event. I look forward to nap times. This is my chance to catch a short nap myself if I'm feeling weary, spend some uninterrupted time with God, and/or accomplish something around the house that is more difficult to do when my little guy is up. Some days, he gives me a whole two hours.

I know nap time is over when I hear the familiar fusses rising from the nursery. After all that sleep, he's hungry! (Did I mention that Benjamin really likes to eat?) I usually have a scrambled egg with cheese and meat mixed in already cooked and cooled with a side of fruit or vegetable. As I strap my son into his high chair again, he uses his "fake fuss" to try and hurry me along. Once his bib is in place, I ask "Benjamin, do you want to *eat*? Tell *Mommy* you want to *eat*." He knows he must make the sign for "eat" before I give him his first bite, and he usually quickly complies. Since transitions tend to be hard for Benjamin, I am sure to warn him when I give him the last bite. Even then, the transition to his cup is often a battle. As soon as my son hears "last bite," his eyes get wide, and he may start to fuss while he still has the food in his mouth. When I offer his cup, he cries and waves his hand in front of him, trying to knock the cup away. "Okay, well you can sit there for a bit, because we're all done eating." Benjamin doesn't seem to have a sense of when he's full, and he will eat as long as food is offered to him. (At restaurants, especially, he is convinced that he should be eating the *entire* time we're there.) After letting him sit for a minute or two, I pick up his drink and offer it to him again. If he still refuses, I will pretend to drink it, which he finds very funny. This usually does the trick, and he will then happily drink, giving a lively commentary of various sounds along the way. When Benjamin decides he's done with his drink, however, he still tends to throw his cup to the ground; a behavior he *knows* gets him into trouble. The discipline most often involves a flick on his cheek along with a stern "No! Do not throw your cup." He scrunches his face as soon as his cup hits the floor, knowing the cheek flick is coming. Upon hearing the "No" from Mommy, though, his little heart usually breaks, and he bursts into tears. He is very sensitive in this way, just as Shawn and I both were as children. This is the typical response, though there have been days when the discipline doesn't seem to phase him in the least.

Benjamin is content to remain in his high chair for a bit after a meal. He chatters away and looks all around or watches what I'm doing in the kitchen. I like that he will sit for a while so his food can settle. Considering his problems with acid reflux, the longer I can keep him upright after a meal, the better. This is a perfect opportunity to vacuum if needed. Benjamin *loves* the vacuum cleaner. When he's particularly excited about something, every muscle in his body tenses; he sticks his legs straight out, his arms are held out in front of him, elbows bent and palms out, and he tightens every muscle in his face for a few seconds. It's quite a sight! He is absolutely fascinated by the vacuum cleaner and watches with wonder as I clean the rug under the table. I often wheel his high chair to the entry of the living room so he can watch me vacuum there as well. I always get cries of protest when the noisy appliance is finally shut off and put away. What a funny guy!

Our afternoons are filled with more play, therapy appointments, or running errands. Benjamin enjoys them all (for the most part). Each week we have either his speech therapist or his child development specialist visit our home to work with him for up to an hour. We receive their services through an early intervention program called Sooner Start that is offered through the local health department. We have been receiving services since he was three months old, and he will be able to receive them for a few more months until his third birthday. What a blessing this program has been! Though Benjamin often fusses while the ladies push him to work, he loves to show off for them too. He knows when he's the center of attention in any given situation, and he is usually more than happy to rise to the occasion. For the last nine months we have also had weekly appointments at the hospital to work with his physical therapist Rebecca. She has helped Benjamin come so far in such a short amount of time. She really knows how to make him work, but she does it in a loving and gentle way, and though he often protests the labor, he seems to like her very much.

Running errands are always a treat for Benjamin because he enjoys car rides and riding in a shopping cart. As soon as I strap him into a cart and start pushing he squeals with delight *at the top of his lungs*, announcing our arrival to the entire store! He puts his head down and watches the floor as we move along or twists himself around in the seat, trying to get a better view of where we're going. He always draws some measure of attention and affection during our outings. Strangers come up to talk to him and pat his hand. I've even had some bold ones come up and kiss him! Benjamin is a people magnet and seems to brighten days wherever we go.

Afternoons go quickly, and 3:30 is the celebrated time when Daddy comes home. A few months after the birth of IHOP-B in June 2011, Shawn took a job at a local middle school as a paraprofessional. He is currently working with a boy who has cerebral palsy and is wheelchair bound. He wanted a job that required less evening time and less administrative energy than he had at his previous position so he could focus more attention on the new church. He really enjoys his job, and we all love that he is home in the afternoon, which is one of Benjamin's prime times. Daddy usually walks in the door while Benjamin is in his high chair, yet again, for a small afternoon snack. "Benjamin, Daddy's home! Where's Daddy?" Benjamin smiles and happily looks to the door. He enjoys playing with Daddy, and his favorite game is to be tossed up in the air. He squeals with delight as Shawn tosses him and catches him over and over. This is definitely *Daddy's* game as Mommy's arms could never handle it!

When it's time for me to work on supper, Benjamin usually has some more time in his Super Stand with a movie. This also gives Shawn and me an opportunity to eat and talk before one of us feeds our son and the other does some cleaning up. If we have the evening at home, we may pull out Benjamin's big yellow ball and sit in a circle in the living room. Benjamin loves balls, especially this one which is almost as big as he is. He stretches out his legs and curls his toes in excitement, squealing and laughing and grinning from ear to ear. He grabs the ball and uses both his arms and legs to hold it in front of him, while he licks his tongue across its surface. Then he pushes the ball to Shawn or me, laughing again. We have so much fun! Sometimes, though, it becomes too much fun for his tired little body to handle, and Benjamin's squeals of delight can quickly turn to fusses and tears if the stimulation becomes too much for him. Cuddles, books, and/or his evening cup of milk can be a good remedy if we get to this point.

A few evenings a week, we are down at our church for worship, prayer, and teaching. Though our sleepy son will often express his discontent as his energy wanes, he absolutely loves music and the presence of God. Our church is small, with a family atmosphere, so Benjamin is free to play on the floor and drink his milk while the evening's activity goes on around him. He often crawls and sits in front of Myong and me as we play guitar. He squeals and dances and sometimes looks in awe at different spots around the room while we worship, as though he's seeing something that is veiled to the rest of us. I am convinced that he sees angels at times.

Benjamin can also bring lightheartedness to our worship services. At a recent prayer gathering he was on the floor in front of us as we played and sang, enthusiastically bobbing his head and legs up and down while lying on his stomach. His joyful motion brought an unexpected release of something not so spiritual, and I soon noticed a strong odor rising from my son. He may be little, but he can produce some very powerful stink! This was of the silent but deadly nature. I knew Myong smelled it too, and before long she burst into laughter, unable to play. I quickly followed suit, and between my giggles I explained to everyone else what had just happened. That got us all going, and soon the room was filled with wonderful, refreshing laughter. Benjamin didn't realize he was the source of it all, but he smiled and laughed and looked around, happy to join in. I was sure that Jesus was laughing right along with us.

By 8:30 pm, our little guy is struggling to keep his eyes open. Whether he's still fighting to stay awake or already asleep, one or both of us will gently lay Benjamin down in his crib for the night and pray a blessing over him. I love to watch his peaceful little face as he drifts off to sleep, and I wonder what will fill his dreams that night. I admire his beautiful features and feel thankful that he's my son. I look forward to the days and years of watching him grow from toddler to boy to adolescent to man, and I wonder what our relationship will look like along the way. I wonder what things will mark his life and personality, and I hope and pray that Jesus is at the center of it all. I look forward to seeing the unique expression of God's heart that Benjamin will bring to the world as his personality unfolds in days and years to come. I look forward to seeing him be who he was created to be. There is so much more I could say about my sweet son, but I hope that my words have at least captured the essence of Benjamin.

Unconditional Love

Even though I had to give him a stern "No" a few minutes ago for throwing his cup, Benjamin crawls towards me, smiling and laughing, eager to climb up into my lap. He is fully confident and fully expectant that he will be received with hugs and kisses. His mind is not on the recent discipline but on the love he knows his mommy has for him. He comes to me at any time of the day, no matter what is happening or who is around, wanting and expecting my attention and affection. . . and he gets it. Benjamin doesn't analyze his behavior over the day to determine whether I will receive him or whether I will hold him at arm's length. He doesn't try to find ways to "earn" back my favor after being disciplined. He approaches me with laughter and with joy, or with tears and the desire for comfort; either way he is confident he will be received with love and acceptance.

This morning Father God ministered to my heart through the simplicity of my sweet son. As I love my son, I get a small glimpse into the heart of a loving God. As I write this, I am listening to the live web stream from the International House of Prayer in Kansas City. The worship team has just broken into spontaneous song. A young woman is singing, "What a Father You are. You never reject us or turn us away. Though our fathers and mothers reject us, You never turn us away." *I'm listening, Daddy! You are speaking to me!* I cannot conceive of ever rejecting my son. Yet I know that my love is still an imperfect love. I also know that there are wounded fathers and mothers in this world who do reject their children, whether intentionally or unintentionally. All too often they are repeating the unhealthy patterns they experienced as children. And though it is my desire to love my child wholeheartedly, I know that in my imperfection, Benjamin will no doubt experience feelings of rejection from me to some degree during his life. There is not a single human relationship immune from mistakes and disappointments.

Father God, though, is a different story. His love is perfect, unconditional, and constant. Love originates in Him and finds its ultimate fulfillment in Him. It does not stand to reason that my love and delight for my son could be greater than the Father's love and delight for me. It does not stand to reason that He would give me affection for "good" behavior and withhold it for "bad" behavior. His heart is always for me; His affection is always extended to me. Like Benjamin, though, I have a part to play. I must be willing to come to Him with simple trust and love, confident that I will be received. I will be loved.

True Value

One recent morning, Shawn didn't have time to pack his lunch before leaving for work, so I called later, offering to run one by the school for him. He gratefully agreed, then called back asking me to bring it by the old high school gym instead of the middle school where he primarily works. It was the weekly practice for the Special Olympics, and students from elementary school through high school would be bussed to the gym to take part in the exercises. Shawn would be there with the young man he works with. His "kiddo" as my husband likes to call him is a great kid with a delightful personality, and I love hearing Shawn's stories about their interactions at school. They make a good team! I was excited that things were timed so perfectly; I had wanted to check out one of the practices since I'd heard about them a few weeks prior. I quickly put together Shawn's lunch, got Benjamin ready, and headed to the car. I couldn't wait to meet Shawn's kiddo and see all the children and teens participating in the practice. I was looking forward to watching Shawn proudly introduce our son to students and staff. I was eager to see how the Special Olympics practice was structured, as we have every intention of encouraging Benjamin to participate when he is old enough. I was confident that I would feel right at home in this setting. After all, I am the parent and primary caregiver for a child with special needs. Speculations can never be proven as reality, however, until they are tested, and I was to be surprised by how I responded.

Benjamin fell asleep in the car shortly before we pulled into the school parking lot. Shawn ran outside to meet us, and since it was cold, he grabbed Benjamin and ran back inside while I followed behind with the stroller, diaper bag, and his lunch. The cold air and sudden motion woke our son from his brief nap, and he was not pleased to be whisked away to an unfamiliar setting when he would rather be sleeping. He was cranky from the start. Shawn's kiddo was waiting for us in his wheelchair right inside. I was happy to meet him and asked playfully, "Are you keeping Shawn in line and making sure he behaves himself?" He laughed and answered softly, "No, he keeps me in line." I liked this young man right from the start, but my heart hurt at seeing firsthand the level of his physical disability. As I held Benjamin in my arms he said, "Sometimes I miss being that small." I was dumbfounded. I managed a laugh and asked, "Do you remember being that small?" He quietly replied, "No," and I wondered what would cause a sixth grade boy to miss the dependency of toddlerhood. I realized, though, that he has experienced very little opportunity for independence in his life due to the limitations of his condition. Dependence on others to assist with his basic needs has been his way of life.

We made our way into the gym, where most of the students were sitting on the bleachers, waiting for their turn to race, one of the first activities of the day. Most of them were excited to see a small child, and many gathered around us inquisitively. Shawn proudly made some introductions and tried to walk around with Benjamin, but by this point our toddler was overwhelmed by all the new people, the noise and unfamiliar environment, and all he wanted was Mommy! I held him and comforted him and tried to answer the students' questions. A teenage girl whose speech indicated her cognitive disability kept insisting on seeing him again. At one point she stated that she wanted to hold Benjamin, but I ignored her request, knowing it would not go well. I didn't want to admit it to myself, but I felt uncomfortable in her presence.

As I looked around the gym, I saw many different levels of disabilities. There were a few other children with Down syndrome; one little boy in particular we had met on more than one occasion. A small number of students were wheelchair bound, some with limited use of their limbs and some completely immobilized. There were some students who had no apparent physical disability, but their speech demonstrated cognitive delay. Due to my son's cries, I had to leave the gym a few times to try and calm him down, but I hoped to be able to watch at least a few of the morning's activities. I was able to watch Shawn's kiddo slowly wheel himself part way across the gym and then around some orange cones that were set out for him. It took him a long time, but the staff and students were cheering him the whole way!

I finally got Benjamin calm enough to sit on the first bleacher right inside the door, but it didn't last long. During the few minutes we had, I watched a couple of the races, as students ran across the gym three at a time. Though most were slow and their movements were awkward, they received a constant flow of cheers and affirmation, and they were clearly enjoying themselves. I was able to the watch the little boy with Down syndrome whom we know race against two other boys, one of whom also has Down syndrome. He ran his little heart out and left the other two boys trailing behind. *Which one will Benjamin be?* I wondered. *Will he thrive in the Special Olympics and athletics, or will his interests center elsewhere?* If he takes after his Daddy, it will be athletics. If he takes after me, it will be the arts. Maybe it will be mix of the two or something else entirely that we haven't even thought of yet!

I felt such an array of emotions as we sat there. I wasn't as prepared as I had thought to see so many different disabilities up close. I thought I would feel at ease and at home, but instead I felt out of place. I know Benjamin has Down syndrome; I witness firsthand the disabilities and delays he faces on a daily basis. However, first and foremost, he is my son. I *know* him, and I am comfortable in knowing him. I did not know these other children, and I was ashamed of the discomfort I felt in their presence. I reflected on how each one was someone's son or daughter, loved and valued (if all is as it should be) just as I love my son. I silently prayed that God would give me eyes to truly see the beautiful people filling the room. I realized that as Benjamin grows, this will become an increasingly familiar community to us. I wrestled some with that reality, a tinge of grief piercing my heart. It was another reminder that life will look different with our son than what we once envisioned. I wondered, *What does it look like to bring the Kingdom of God to these ones?* I want my heart to truly love them.

It didn't take long before Benjamin was wailing again, so we said our goodbyes to Shawn and headed home. I reflected in the car as we drove, and I've reflected more over the days since this experience. I've had many thoughts. I've thought about the value and beauty of each human life. We live in a culture where appearance and personal achievement are highly prized and sought after, worshipped even. In the midst of such propaganda and pressure, do we remember to simply value people? Benjamin may never take first place in a race or any other event. He may come in dead last, even at the Special Olympics. Whether he's first, last, or one of the many in-between places, will that alter the level of pride I have for my son or the value he holds in my heart? Absolutely not! While there is a healthy place of pride for our children's accomplishments, I don't want that pride to ever be based on how he "measures up" to those around him. I want Benjamin to know that his dad and I are full of pride for him, simply because he's our son. I want to cheer him on with enthusiasm as he runs this marathon called life, encouraging him to be who he was created to be.

I also thought about how much needless emotional and mental energy I waste when I critique whether or not I'm "measuring up" to those around me. My Heavenly Father doesn't compare me to others, so why am I so quick to compare myself? He loves me simply because I am His. I thought about how much I can learn about God's Kingdom from the special needs community, a community comprised of so many unique individuals, each with their own beauty to offer the world. I want to see Jesus in the faces of the ones the world may consider unlovely. I want to be reminded of Him in the ones the world may cast aside as forgotten. I want to give and receive His unconditional love that is never based on performance and is only experienced through relationship. I want to value what He values.

Mr. Mobile!

It felt like one of the longest waits of my life. I remember when Shawn's dad D.J. came to visit shortly after Benjamin's first homecoming from the hospital. Our son was just barely two months old. His heart surgery was only days away. Before reluctantly leaving to head back to Minnesota, D.J. said, "He'll probably be crawling around when we see you at Christmas." Knowing that our little son would only be seven months old by then and that he would experience developmental delays, I responded, "Well, maybe not this Christmas, but definitely by next Christmas!" After all, Benjamin would be nineteen months old by that point. I couldn't fathom him seeing his first birthday before he was crawling. However, faster than I thought possible, his first birthday arrived, and not only was Benjamin not crawling yet, he wasn't even able to sit up without moderate assistance. We purchased him a Bumbo seat and used it as long as we could, but he was really too big for it in the first place. It's not designed for a one year old. One year olds are typically long past the need for that type of intervention and many are toddling around.

I remember our first few visits to the Down Syndrome Association of Tulsa meetings during Benjamin's first year. We saw a couple of two year olds who were up and walking around. I remember thinking, "That's not so bad. At least we have a better idea of when he should meet his milestones." However, we were not anticipating all of the medical complications Benjamin would face in his first few years. By the time we had reached our son's first birthday he had experienced premature birth, extended respiratory distress, jaundice, kidney failure (all those just within the first week of life), open heart surgery, double hernia surgery, infantile spasm seizures, an MRI of his brain which required general anesthesia, ear tube surgery, and the diagnosis of permanent mild/moderate hearing loss the literal day before his birthday. In the following year and three months he would also undergo two eye surgeries and his short stint with glasses. Besides the Down syndrome, premature birth, and open heart surgery, the seizures in particular resulted in significant developmental delays for our son. We are so incredibly thankful that Jesus healed him of these, as in time they could have caused permanent brain damage and even more extensive delays. We are still praying for the full restoration of what Benjamin lost during those months.

On top of this extensive list Benjamin was born with very low muscle tone, and he was born very big. Low muscle tone is a common trait associated with Down syndrome. We have been told by more than one therapist that Benjamin's muscle tone is on the low end of low. Upon feeling his legs for the first time, one therapist remarked, "You want to make sure we *know* that you have Down syndrome!" I feel like I should interject a story here with this in mind: When Benjamin was in the hospital following his open heart surgery, Shawn and I visited a church where we had previously attended some weekend conferences. However, it was our first time to attend a regular Sunday morning service. As a gesture of love and welcome, first-time visitors are invited to go to a separate room at the back of the church after the service in order to receive personal prayer ministry. Shawn and I were desperate for encouragement. During this ministry time, one of the two ladies who were praying for us kept hearing the phrase "strong trunk" run through her mind. She had no idea what it meant. We knew exactly what it meant! We had already been told by medical professionals that it would be critical for Benjamin to develop good *trunk* support because most of the body's movement is dependent on its mid-section. We have held on to that word for a long time! *

Anyway, back to his size... Benjamin weighed 7 pounds, 6 ounces when he was born, in contrast to an average birth weight of 5 pounds for a full-term infant with Down syndrome. Ever since then he has been at the very top of the Down syndrome growth charts or above them. While his bigger size may have benefited him in some ways as a newborn, his size combined with his low muscle tone have created another hindrance for mobility.

When Benjamin was fourteen months old, he was finally able to maintain a sitting position by himself. We were thrilled! However, he was not able to get himself in and out of this position, and he was so used to being dependent on us for most things, that he wouldn't even reach for a toy that was placed a short distance away from him. He was able to play with many of his toys more effectively, but his personal independence was still very limited. Shawn and I worked at trying to help him crawl, but it felt like he fought us every step of the way. Benjamin was never really a fan of tummy time, and that's a nice way of saying it! He was primarily confined to his back for his first three months of life because of his medical conditions, and by that point he wanted nothing to do with being on his stomach. We tried positioning him to bear down weight on his hands and wrists, but he would just bend his elbows, collapse on the floor and fill the room with his cries of anger. Our attempts to position him on his knees created very similar results.

One day I saw an online video of a mother using a string of Christmas lights to motivate her son with Down syndrome to crawl. So, we pulled out the Christmas lights. Benjamin was very intrigued by them, but he did not appreciate the process that would follow. I would kneel on the floor and keep them just out of his reach while Shawn would bend one of Benjamin's knees and then the other, helping him push off Daddy's leg with his little foot to propel him forward inch by inch on his belly. Sometimes the lights were enough of a distraction to go a few feet. It didn't take long, though, for Benjamin to have our little scheme figured out, and he wanted nothing to do with the game anymore.

Before we knew it, Benjamin's second Christmas had come and gone, and there was still no indication that we would be crawling any time soon. I cried many tears over this sobering reality. Some days the grief and anger would rise up so strong inside of me. Why did my son have to have so much stacked against him? Why did this all have to be so hard for him? He didn't look like an infant, but developmentally he was still very much a baby. It felt like I was getting asked questions all the time: "Is he crawling yet?" (There was one senior citizen at The Salvation Army who literally asked this almost *every* week). "When is he supposed to crawl?" I felt so helpless at this point, and people's questions of concern only seemed to fuel my frustration. At the same time I was being faced with the reality that babies who had been *conceived* during my son's first year were up and crawling around, even pulling up to stand, while my child was still just rolling around on the floor. I tried to step back from time to time and regain perspective, "He will crawl one day," I would tell myself. "He will not only crawl, but he will walk and talk and play. This is only a season." Oh, but how long would this season last!

Shortly before Benjamin's second birthday we started taking him to Rebecca for additional therapy. From day one we started working hard to help him sit up independently. A few weeks after his birthday, our son finally made the breakthrough of being able to get in and out of a sitting position, and a whole new world of freedom and independence opened up to him. It was thrilling in a very bittersweet way. When I had expected a toddling toddler, I had a very big boy pushing with all his might to get himself upright, but I was so proud of him! Soon he was doing it so naturally that it was hard to imagine the months of struggle that had preceded this new milestone. I continued to pray as I had for the last year and a half that my son would soon learn to crawl.

By this point Benjamin had also started pushing up some on his hands and arms, but he didn't know how to get his knees under him. He was becoming more tolerant of having assistance in this area as we practiced holding him on hands and knees or placing him in a tall kneeling position up against low furniture with a favorite toy as motivation. We could tell he was gaining strength, and we were so encouraged! Overall he was a happier boy, and his personality was emerging more and more.

Then one typical morning, (July 18, 2011 to be exact) Shawn and I were sitting in the living room sipping coffee and reading our Bibles as Benjamin played on the floor. Suddenly, using his arms and one leg, Benjamin started moving himself forward on his belly to reach a toy that he couldn't get to otherwise. At first we could hardly believe what we were seeing! Our son was FINALLY using a form of crawling! It was so amazing yet so surreal. We had waited and waited and waited for this moment, and it was finally happening! In the days, weeks, and months that followed, he became faster and more proficient at his little army crawl. He was a different child! His fussiness subsided bit by bit as he took more self-initiative and embraced his new independence. It was so exciting to see. We continued to work on getting him up on hands and knees and holding him at his hips to help him rock back and forth, which became one of his favorite games. I would say, "Hey, Benjamin, let's rock!" He would start to get up onto hands and knees and rock back and forth with my assistance (which he started needing less and less) as I would chant, "Rock, rock, rock! Rock, rock, rock! Rockin' baby Benjamin. Rock, rock, rock!" He loved it.

By his third Christmas, he had started crawling a "step" or two on his hands and knees before reverting back to his stomach. He also started pushing up on his hands and feet into a bear crawling position. He loved and still loves to hold his head upside down and look between his legs. It's adorable! Then in January 2012, he began to crawl everywhere, and he is fast. He is much braver than when he first started crawling, and he loves to explore the whole house. It's difficult to keep him contained in one room for very long. He has places to go and things to get into! As with all of his previous developmental breakthroughs, Benjamin is crawling so naturally now that it's hard to remember what a long and hard process it was to get to this point. There's not a day that goes by that my heart is not warmed at seeing my son crawl around, even when I wish he'd sit still just for a little while.

During the months and years of waiting, some people would try to make me feel better by saying, "Oh, just you wait. When he does start crawling you'll be sorry." Those comments never made me feel better. I would usually respond, "No, I am more than ready for him to crawl. I will celebrate when he crawls, even if it means more work." There has never been the fraction of a second that I've felt sorry that my son is crawling. Yes, I have had to be on my toes more, but it is worth every moment! The unavoidable "inconveniences" of a busy baby is nothing compared to the pain of his extended delays.

Benjamin has just recently started pulling up to stand at furniture. The familiar emotions of longing for my son to crawl have transferred to a longing to see him walk. At the time I write this, Benjamin's third birthday is just around the corner. He is currently at least three feet tall and weighs over 30 pounds. While his crawling has saved me from having to carry him everywhere, I still have to carry him a lot. I am a tired mama! At the first baby shower we had for Benjamin, we received two small picture frames, one that reads "First Smile" and the other that reads "First Step." They are both on display in his room, one with a sweet picture of Benjamin smiling at his daddy and the other sitting empty, waiting for the day it can be filled. I remind myself that, just like the crawling and so many other milestones that we have worked and worked for, Benjamin will walk, and I believe that he will walk well in time. As with the crawling, the wait feels long and hard, but it's encouraging to know that it's only temporary. Keep moving forward, Benjamin! Mommy and Daddy (and many others) are cheering you the whole way!

In early 2014 a temporary therapist we had not worked with before made multiple comments about Benjamin's strong trunk. The word we held on to for five years has finally come to pass!

Help that Hurts

We have all had the experience of seeing a loved one or acquaintance in deep emotional pain. I believe we have all wished we could find the right words to say to ease their suffering. I believe many of us have also felt discomfort when encountering another's grief up close, wanting an escape from the awkwardness of the situation. I have been on this end of relationship many times, and I know I have been too quick to share words that seemed to only hit the ground, even though my intentions were good. However, through my experiences since Benjamin's birth of being the one in pain, I believe I have learned a bit more about what truly helps as opposed to "help" that hurts.

As I have written elsewhere, Shawn and I have been the recipients of incredible support and encouragement since we began our journey of parenting a child with special needs. We have been truly blessed through the genuine love and investment of others in our lives, and we will always be thankful. However, I now want to focus on the "help" that hasn't been so helpful. My motive in writing this piece is not to point the finger or be critical of others, but instead to create awareness on a very sensitive issue. Where to begin….

I have realized more and more since my son's birth that many people tend to hold a "rose-colored glasses" view of having a child with Down syndrome. Shawn and I have cringed inside time and time again as friends or even strangers have made comments such as, "God only gives these children to special people." "Oh, they're all such little *angels*." "God knew you could handle it." Do I believe that Benjamin is a gift? Absolutely—just as I believe that every child born is a gift, regardless of the circumstances. I highly value human life, and I cherish my son. However, I do not feel that children with disabilities are only given to *special* people who "can handle it." All around the world, children with Down syndrome and other special needs are abandoned to orphanages and institutions. Their parents didn't feel *special* and instead rejected the very life they had created. I have heard that in our nation ninety percent or more of women who receive a prenatal diagnosis of Down syndrome choose to abort. There is no rosy notion here but a devastating reality.

As to the sentiment that all people with Down syndrome are like angels, such comments carry a bit of a sting as well. Benjamin is a delightful little boy, and I love watching his personality blossom. However, his love or happiness as an individual is not dependent on the fact that he carries an extra chromosome. He will be shaped by relationships and life experiences just like we all are, and he will be his own person with good days and bad days, joys and sorrows. We once had a friend tell us about a grown man who had Down syndrome that she had encountered at a restaurant. He was an outgoing individual, making conversation with many people. She told us, "I thought, 'That's Benjamin!'" I knew she meant well, but it was upsetting that my son's personhood was being directly linked to his disability, even if it was in a flattering way. We intend to raise him to value people and to walk in love, but we will not assume that his chromosomal condition will ensure his emotional disposition! To the same measure that he can be happy and loving he can also be angry and frustrated. He is a human being with a full range of emotions.

When we've been told that God gave us Benjamin because He knew we could handle it, I want to laugh. We are not somehow immune to pain and disappointment, and it has only been His grace and His strength that have enabled us to walk through both. The underlying message I have felt from such comments has been, "I'm glad it's you and not me. God knows *I* couldn't handle it!" Now I realize that this attitude is not true of everyone, but I hope that I'm making the clear point that having a child with special needs should not be romanticized.

Another way we have experienced "help" that hurts has been the sense that others are reluctant to acknowledge our pain while being quick to give pat answers. Sometimes we have felt that our pain is not acceptable to others; maybe it makes them uncomfortable, so they give us cheery responses that only seem to undermine what we are feeling. While the intentions may be good, the effects are disheartening. One example has been the grief we have experienced over Benjamin's developmental delays. Many times I have opened my heart to another in this matter, only to receive prompt replies such as, "But he's doing so good!" "Oh, well he'll get there!" "Yeah, but he's so cute!" I've even heard such things as, "When he does start (*fill in the blank*), then you'll be sorry." I know that my son is doing well; no one is prouder of him than his parents. I know that "he'll get there," but it doesn't erase the pain that he's not "there" yet. I think he's the cutest little boy in the world, but that doesn't diminish my disappointments over his challenges. I have NEVER been sorry when Benjamin has reached a new milestone. Each one is an occasion for much celebration and thanksgiving. Few people truly grasp the amount of work, tears, frustration, and prayer that have been invested into each one.

As I have experienced misdirected "help" over these past few years, I have realized more and more how many times I have been guilty of doing the same. My hope and prayer is that my experiences are teaching me to be more compassionate and sensitive when I encounter pain in others. I have learned that silence can sometimes be the greatest help. Those that have been willing to simply *listen* to me share the pain of my heart without trying to *fix* me have been the most comforting of all. There are often no right words to say when someone is hurting. Listen to me, cry with me, offer a hug, pray with me, and trust Jesus to heal my heart. He is the Great Physician. His words are the words that bring life and healing. Sometimes He may give you words to say, but be sensitive to His leading in this area. As I've written previously, early in the journey we had two friends come to us with the gentle exhortation to set our hearts before Jesus to receive healing. They didn't speak many words, only the words they felt God had given them. I also know that they prayed for us before ever releasing those words to us. As we took their advice to heart, we received a deeper measure of healing than a multitude of well-intentioned words could have ever offered to us. I think we should all seek to follow the wisdom of James 1:19 to *"...be swift to hear, slow to speak..."* This will truly help!

You Heard What I Said!

On the morning of May 21, 2010, Mom and I drove Benjamin to the Diagnostic Neurophysiology building in Tulsa for his scheduled sedated ABR (Auditory Brainstem Response) procedure. (That was all a mouthful, I know!) His first birthday was the very next day, and I could think of a hundred things I would rather be doing. Our son's first year had been full of so many hospital stays, doctor visits, and medical procedures, however, that I had pretty much come to accept them as a normal part of life. Whether the results were good or bad, I was hoping that we would finally get some concrete answers that day about Benjamin's hearing.

During his bout with infantile spasm seizures, he had a routine hearing test with his audiologist, a recommended intervention for children with Down syndrome, as around 50-60% of this population suffers from some degree of hearing loss. There are three possible types of hearing loss:

1. *Conductive*—referring to a build of fluid in the middle ears that creates interference with the conduction of sound vibrations in the middle ear
2. *Sensorineural*— referring to a damage to bones and/or nerves in the inner ear that affects the transfer of sound from the inner ear to the auditory nerve
3. *Mixed*—referring to the presence of both types of hearing loss

One common characteristic for children with Down syndrome is small ear canals, which can often increase the problem of fluid retention in the inner ear and lead to chronic ear infections. This in turn can cause conductive hearing loss. The good news about this type of loss is that it is not permanent. The surgical insertion of ear tubes to allow the inner ear to drain is often all it takes to return hearing to normal levels. Sensorineural hearing loss, on the other hand, is not curable. In young children with this type of hearing loss, the damage to the inner ear is often present at birth. It is the most common type of permanent hearing loss, and hearing aids are the most common solution to help improve hearing ability.

I do not want to sound like I'm writing out of a textbook, but I believe some basic information about the types of hearing loss will enable me to share our story with more credibility and meaning. When Benjamin had his first hearing test in February 2010, the results were not good. He was not responsive to the level the audiologist wanted to see. Behavioral hearing tests are difficult with small children and leave a definite margin for error, but they can assist in determining if there may be a problem. We tested again in March, but the results had not improved. In daily life Benjamin was not as responsive as we would like either. The seizures had definitely played a part in this, but we couldn't assume they were the only reason for the delays. The audiologist recommended us to an Ear, Nose, and Throat specialist (ENT) for the purpose of having ear tubes inserted. Our hope was that Benjamin's potential hearing loss was conductive, and we would see an improvement after having the simple surgery, which he had at the end of March. It was a simple out-patient procedure, but we still dreaded our son having to be sedated again for another operation. Hospital settings had become all too familiar. Our ENT was very helpful and kind, but he told us before surgery that Benjamin's ear canals were some of the smallest he had ever seen, even for a child with Down syndrome. He could not guarantee that he would be successful in inserting the ear tubes. Thankfully, though, the surgery was a success, but he told us that he saw very little fluid in our son's ears. We still hoped we would begin to see improvement in Benjamin's responsiveness to sound, but this was not the case.

For this reason, I found myself in Tulsa the day before my son's birthday for the ABR test. In this particular test, the child must be asleep for the entire procedure. Benjamin was given oral medication to make him drowsy, and once he was asleep, the audiologist prepped him for the procedure while Mom and I waited in a small office across the hall. She told us the test itself would take around an hour for each ear, so we settled in for the long wait. During an ABR, small electrodes are connected to the child's scalp and a small microphone is placed in the ear canal. A computer then charts the brain's responses to sounds sent directly into the ear. It is the most accurate hearing test for small children.

I don't remember how long we waited in that little room, but I do remember that the time seemed to drag by. Mom had flown in for a visit earlier in the week, and I was grateful for her company. It was an early morning test, and we were both sleepy. I was anxious as well, wanting answers, but afraid of what the answers might be. When the ABR was finally finished, the audiologist came to talk with us. To my dismay, she gave the report I did not want to hear. According to her test results, Benjamin had sensorineural hearing loss, mild in his right ear and moderate in his left. I tried to process what she was saying and asked if there was any chance his hearing would ever improve. She gently explained that his loss was permanent, and there was a possibility it could get worse over time. I felt numb. She recommended that we have him fitted for hearing aids soon, an intervention he would need for life. An excerpt of the official report reads as follows:

IMPRESSION: *The above test battery is consistent with a moderately sloping most likely sensorineural hearing loss in the left ear, and a mildly sloping most likely SN loss in the right. (Bone conduction thresholds abnormal).*

RECOMMEND:

1. *Medical management of blocked vs extruded PE tubes au.*
2. *Bilateral hearing aid evaluation.*
3. *Close monitoring of hearing levels due to the possibility of progressive hearing loss.*

My heart sank. Did this have to be the hallmark for the end of Benjamin's first year? Hadn't he been through more than enough already? Our little boy had experienced more medically in one year's time than some people do over a lifetime. How much more would we have to deal with?

The following day we celebrated our son's first birthday with family and friends. Overall, the party went well, and we were all able to enjoy ourselves. I had some anxiety leading up to the party, however. I wanted everything to be perfect, and little details were blown up big in my emotions, making me feel tense and irritable. Shawn was encouraging me to relax and just enjoy myself, but I was struggling. Inwardly I was chastising myself for behaving this way. Today was supposed to be a day of celebration, and I wanted to enjoy it. I soon realized the root of my intensity. Ever since Benjamin's birth, I had felt so out of control of so many things. I felt so helpless to be able to help my son on numerous occasions. His first birthday party felt to me like something I finally had a measure of control over; it was something special I could do for him, and I wanted it to be perfect since so many things had been less than perfect during this first year. Recognizing where I was helped me to relax some and regain perspective. The important thing was that we enjoy Benjamin and enjoy our loved ones celebrating with us. The other details were secondary.

Within a few weeks Benjamin was fitted for hearing aids, and they arrived less than two weeks later. On June 17, I drove my small son to Tulsa again, this time to The Scholl Center for

Communication Disorders, to pick them up. I found it ironic that this day marked the one year anniversary of Benjamin's homecoming from the NICU. Who knew how much one year could hold! The audiologists at The Scholl Center were very kind and showed me how to insert and care for the new hearing aids. I was thankful that everything appeared to be quite simple. Benjamin didn't put up the fuss I thought he would when they were first fitted in his ears. We were given a set of small fabric casings that slipped over each hearing aid and were attached to a string that could be clipped to the back of Benjamin's shirt. This would help to ensure that the hearing aids wouldn't be lost if they fell out (or he pulled them out). I was also advised that a small strip of toupee tape on the back of each hearing aid would help to hold it in place against my son's head without any discomfort for him. In the weeks and months that followed, we discovered that we preferred to use the tape for day to day life at home and the casings for outings. Benjamin had two more hearing tests, one with and one without the hearing aids. With the hearing aids in place, his hearing tested close to normal levels. Shawn and I were so encouraged!

The drive home from Tulsa that day was a new experience. It was close to rush hour, so there was extra sound and activity on the highway. Benjamin screamed the whole way through Tulsa. I realized that he'd never heard the amplified sounds of heavy traffic before, and the new sensation scared him. I felt sad for his distress but excited that he was clearly hearing more!

Over the next few weeks, Benjamin adjusted to the hearing aids better than we could have imagined. It was obvious that they were helping him, and he liked wearing them. He was still a long way from crawling at this point, but was rolling all over the place, creating a challenge for keeping the aids in place. However, it was rare that he actually pulled them out himself. If the molds weren't fitting quite right, and he was getting a lot of feedback he'd take them out; otherwise, they seemed to become a part of him. Shawn and I noticed a marked difference in his responsiveness, as did his therapist. Overall he was more alert and a happier little guy. We were so thankful!

Since children grow so quickly, Benjamin had to have new molds cast about every four months. He never did appreciate this procedure. Whenever the time came to replace the molds, I was able to choose from a variety of colors, but I always stuck with some shade of blue, though one time we did a blue and white swirl. I thought the blue brought out Benjamin's eyes. For the hearing aids themselves, which would last for at least a few years, I had chosen a neutral color that was the mix between a tan and a light brown. We had a sheet of hearing aid stickers with which to decorate them, and I usually changed Benjamin's stickers whenever he received new ear molds. I always wondered what his preferences would be for colors and stickers when he was old enough to choose himself.

The hearing aids quickly became a normal part of life, though Shawn and I never stopped asking God for a miracle in our son's hearing ability. We had already witnessed Benjamin's healing from seizures, and we knew we had a miracle baby. Whenever there was the opportunity for others to pray for his hearing, we eagerly sought it out. If we went to listen to a guest minister speak, we took Benjamin up to receive prayer. When we shared his amazing testimony of healing from seizures at the One Thing Conference at the International House of Prayer in Kansas City, the whole audience joined in praying for him. He was prayed for at our own prayer gatherings on a consistent basis. And, of course, we prayed over him in our home all the time. However, Benjamin couldn't tell us if anything was happening to him, so we just trusted that time would tell.

In the fall of 2011, we had a bad string of ear molds. One pair never fit well, and Benjamin wouldn't keep them in, so we had them replaced. The next pair wasn't much better. During the intervals of waiting for the new molds to come in, there wasn't much point in trying to keep his hearing aids in because he was so quick to pull them out. I had hoped that a new set would be in before we left for Minnesota to spend Christmas with Shawn's family, but they didn't make it back on time, so we left for our trip without even bothering to pack the hearing aids.

When we finally received his new molds in January, we still seemed to be having problems. Benjamin had always enjoyed wearing his hearing aids; why was he suddenly fighting them so much? He would cry every time I tried to put them in. By this point it had been a few months since he had worn them consistently, and I wrestled with feelings of guilt over this fact. However, during those few months Shawn and I were noticing a new level of responsiveness in Benjamin even without the hearing aids in place. For instance, if he was sitting in his high chair and the coffee pot on the other side of the kitchen started to brew, he would turn around and look for the source of the sound. He would respond to our voices spoken softly, even if he wasn't looking at us when we spoke. He was turning towards various noises more and more in general. Our hopes began to rise.

I brought these things to the attention of our audiologist and requested to have some more hearing tests done. She wanted to stick with behavioral hearing tests at first, but we found out during one of the first attempts that Benjamin had a build-up of ear wax in his ear. She recommended we have it cleaned out. At the end of January 2012 we had an appointment with the ENT, who extracted some large pieces of wax from inside Benjamin's ears. One of his ear tubes had already fallen out previously, and the remaining tube came out with a glob of wax. However, since Benjamin never had chronic ear infections, the ENT didn't feel it was necessary to replace the tubes again.

Our audiologist works at multiple sites, and she happened to be at our ENT's office that day, so she performed a behavioral hearing test on Benjamin with his freshly cleaned ears. She was surprised and excited by the results. He was responding in the low normal range, *without his hearing aids.* The next step now was to schedule another ABR.

On March 1, Shawn and I drove to The Scholl Center for what ended up being round one of Benjamin's ABR testing. Since sedation was not going to be used for this testing, we had to try to plan the appointment close to nap time and hope that he would sleep long enough to test his ears. We were taken back to a little room decorated like a nursery with the lights dimmed. I held Benjamin on my lap in an oversized recliner as the young woman who would be performing the test began prepping our son for the procedure. She was very kind, interning for what was the last semester of her Ph.D. program. Benjamin, however, did not appreciate her at all and screamed and twisted around in my arms as she hooked up the electrodes to his head and inserted the microphone in his ear. Now the challenge was to get him to sleep. She wisely stepped out for a while, so I could soothe him. Shawn sat across the room from me, trying to stay awake himself as I sang "Twinkle, Twinkle Little Star" for what felt like fifty times. My angry toddler finally fell asleep in my arms. The test could begin. Each ear required an hour for testing, so we knew it wasn't likely that Benjamin would stay asleep long enough to test both ears. I didn't think my arms could hold out that long either. As my son slept and the computer monitor charted what looked to me like nothing more than squiggly lines, we either chatted some with the young audiologist, with whom we found we had some mutual acquaintances, or we sat in silence. My arms were aching and my stomach was growling before it was all said and done.

Shortly after the test on Benjamin's right ear was completed he began to stir, and he was not happy to wake up to the same surroundings he'd fallen asleep in. We scheduled a second appointment for two weeks later to test his left ear. The audiologist was a bit hesitant to talk to us about her observations from the test. We had already told her our son's story and were honest about our hopes that God had healed him. We knew from our conversation that she was a Christian, and we knew she didn't want us to be disappointed. She said that she really wanted to run the test results by her supervisor for a second opinion. However, she did admit that from what she was seeing so far, she could not find any indication of hearing loss in his right ear! We were thrilled!

Since we were already in Tulsa, and Shawn had taken the day off of work, we decided to take some time to enjoy ourselves while we were there. We headed to one of our favorite restaurants, Panera Bread, for a celebration lunch. (Benjamin loves their macaroni and cheese.) After enjoying a delicious meal, topped off with a steaming cup of hazelnut coffee for Shawn and me and juice for Benjamin, we headed for La Fortune Park. It was a perfect day to be outdoors, and the park with its lovely walking trail, duck pond, and playground equipment, was the perfect place to be. We enjoyed the sunshine, the scenery, and some quality family time as we rejoiced in our son's good report.

Two weeks later we found ourselves back at The Scholl Center to have Benjamin's left ear tested. The young audiologist quickly confirmed the results of the previous test: her supervisor had looked everything over and agreed that it looked perfectly normal! We could hardly wait for what this day's test would reveal, especially since his left ear was the one with the greater level of hearing loss. As anticipated, Benjamin put up quite a fight again before finally falling asleep in my arms, but he eventually gave up, and the hour-long test began. The audiologist was cautious again not to give us a concrete answer without running the results by her supervisor, but she did say that from what she could tell, his left ear was showing either normal hearing or only a very mild loss, a huge improvement from the moderate loss he was originally diagnosed with. We left rejoicing in God's goodness and power demonstrated in Benjamin's life!

On March 20, the first day of spring, the audiologist called us to confirm that report: normal hearing in both ears! There was no concrete explanation for it, either. Over the phone she admitted to me what we already knew to be true, "It could be a miracle." An excerpt from the official report reads as follows:

History: *Parents have noticed that Benjamin seems to be responding better at home while not wearing his hearing aids. A diagnostic ABR...from 5/21/2010 showed a moderately sloping, most likely sensorineural, hearing loss in the left ear and a mildly sloping, most likely sensorineural, hearing loss in the right ear.*

Impression: *Tympanometry was consistent with normal middle ear function bilaterally. Diagnostic ABR results were consistent with normal hearing sensitivity in the left ear. ABR results from 3/1/2012 were consistent with normal hearing sensitivity in the right ear.*

Recommendations: *1) Discontinue bilateral hearing aid use. 2) Seek ear specific behavioral thresholds to confirm ABR results. 3) Continue speech-language therapy.*

Since receiving confirmation of this miracle in Benjamin's hearing, we have shared his testimony with many people. The responses have been mixed. Some have quickly rejoiced with us, believing that our God is a miracle-working God. Others, however, have been skeptical. Some have wondered if Benjamin was misdiagnosed with hearing loss in the first place. I can assure you, he had hearing loss, and he no longer does! A friend of ours who is a licensed speech therapist assured us that ABR test results don't lie. Testing aside, Benjamin's changes in behavior over the past two years related to his hearing are proof enough. A few people have wondered if his ear canals have grown big enough to allow him to hear better. I want to laugh at this one. His ear canals are still so tiny his pediatrician has a difficult time seeing anything when he examines them. When Benjamin was first diagnosed, we were never given any hope that his hearing could improve as he grew. Quite the contrary, we were told it could deteriorate.

Jesus said, *"Assuredly, I say to you, whoever does not receive the kingdom of God as a little child will by no means enter it,"* (Mark 10:15). Jesus also taught His followers to pray, *"Your kingdom come. Your will be done on earth as it is in heaven,"* (Matthew 6:10). There is no hearing loss in heaven. We prayed and others prayed that what was true in heaven would be done on earth in our son's ears, and God heard our prayers. I don't know when or how He healed Benjamin's ears, I just know that He did. You heard what I said!

Treasures in Darkness

Before Benjamin was ever conceived, a spiritual mentor in our lives told us she felt like God had showed her that when we had our first child there would be a struggle of some sort, but the Lord would bring a testimony through it all. She didn't have a clear sense of what this would mean, and neither did we. I'm so thankful that God doesn't tell us everything all at once. Our idea of a struggle looked like a bump in the road compared to the mountains we came up against when our son was born. If we had known ahead of time all that we would face upon Benjamin's birth, I would have had a hard time believing we could make it through. I know the Holy Spirit will reveal to us different things about the future as we ask Him and wait on Him in prayer, but His desire is that we would always depend on Him in the present and trust Him with the future.

When our struggles arrived there was fear and there was shaking, but we never fell past the point of being able to get up again. In our weakest moments we have realized that Jesus has been carrying us in His arms. He has been and continues to be so faithful to sustain us and walk us through. We have and continue to experience the truth of God's Word in 2 Corinthians 12:9…

And He said to me, "My grace is sufficient for you, for My strength is made perfect in weakness…"

We are also learning more the truth of Philippians 4:13…

I can do all things through Christ who strengthens me.

The amazing thing is that, not only are we making it through, but we are emerging from our experiences with a deeper trust in and love for Jesus than ever before. He has planted things deep inside of us through this journey that can never be taken away! He is giving us beauty in exchange for our ashes.

And we know that all things work together for good to those who love God, to those who are called according to His purpose, (Romans 8:28).

I believe there are some treasures that can only be mined in darkness. However, we have to be willing to look for them and be open to receive them. When faced with trials we can choose to simply grit our teeth and try to make it through (sometimes getting stuck along the way), or we can choose to keep moving forward and come out with something beautiful and valuable, made possible only by the grace of God. I believe this is the dividing line between tragedy and triumph. I don't want to miss the treasure to be discovered!

I will give you the treasures of darkness and hidden riches of secret places, that you may know that I, the Lord, Who called you by your name, am the God of Israel, (Isaiah 45:3).

All I've Known is Holland

On July 2, 2012, I stood in our bathroom at 5:00 a.m. with heart pounding as I waited for the results to read on the pregnancy test strip. My heart nearly pounded out of my chest a moment later when the positive sign was revealed! In a state of shock I went and woke up Shawn, who was too groggy at first for the information to register. When he was able to take in what I was saying, he too was shocked and thrilled. After a year and a half of waiting, it felt surreal. We really are going to have another baby!

After rejoicing with me, Shawn drifted back to sleep, but I knew I would not be able to. Instead I went out to the living room to worship, pray, and reflect on this sudden change in our lives. I had known disappointment after disappointment while trying to conceive a second child. The longing had become so intense that it was beginning to consume me. In May the Lord gently put His finger in that very vulnerable place and asked me to lay my desire on the altar. The desire to have children is a good thing in and of itself, but I was so focused on my longing that it was distracting me from my walk with God. He desires that there be no other loves before Him because He created us for relationship with Himself, and He knows that no other love can fully satisfy our hearts. So, in His love, He asked me to surrender my dream for another baby to Him, stop trying to make something happen, and just focus on knowing Him more. With a trembling heart I said "yes," not knowing the fullness of what my yes would require, but knowing that I want to live my life in the center of His will. The "yes" had to be reaffirmed every time the longing arose and sought to overtake my emotions, often multiple times a day. It was both a painful and liberating process. In the midst of the uncertainty and tears of surrender, a new peace descended on my heart. My prayer of "Lord, open my womb," had become "Lord, may Your will be done."

Considering this recent journey He had taken me on, I had no expectation that I would be getting pregnant any time soon. So when my period was late and I was noticing some other unusual symptoms, I tried to not get my hopes up that this was a sign of pregnancy and took the test to rule out the possibility. I was shocked that so soon after I surrendered the desires of my heart to Jesus, He granted me those very desires. I feel like I am living in Psalm 37:4, *"Delight yourself also in the Lord, and He shall give you the desires of your heart."*

As I write this I am entering the tenth week of my pregnancy, and already this one feels different. I am more tired this time, which stands to reason as I did not have a small child to care for the first time around! The queasiness is 24/7 instead of off and on. My "baby bump" is emerging much more rapidly even though I've only gained a pound so far. There isn't the clear sense of whether or not we're having a boy or a girl like we had with Benjamin. Also, this one *just feels different*; I don't have language to describe how or why. The reality that I may finally be taking a trip to "Italy" is growing inside me more and more. Yet all I've known is "Holland."

In some ways I feel like I will have to learn to be a parent all over again. The slower pace of Holland is what I'm familiar with. Every stage of Benjamin's development has been so extended, and every new milestone has required so much work. Currently, he is three years and two months old yet is still operating developmentally like a ten- to twelve-month old. Picturing the much faster pace of Italy is both thrilling and a bit intimidating. I can only imagine Shawn's and my wonder as our next baby seems to effortlessly reaches milestones in his or her first year that Benjamin did not reach until his second or third year after months and months of intervention. I can picture joy in watching our next child's development speed by as well as grief as we remember just how hard Benjamin had to work for the same things.

Though I will be required to have another C-section (most hospitals in Oklahoma will not allow a natural delivery after a prior C-section), my heart is thrilled at the prospect of being able to see my baby right after delivery and being able to hold and nurse my child within a few hours. I am in awe of the thought of being able to bring a healthy baby home at the time of my release from the hospital. I know that this experience is the norm, but for so long it has felt like a distant dream! I also realize that I don't have a clear idea of what the first few months with a newborn are really like. Benjamin was so weak from the holes in his heart that he slept away the majority of his first two months, one of those months confined to the NICU. During his first month home he rarely woke me up to feed him; instead, I had to wake him up to eat. While I know that every child is different and brings his or her own unique experience, I have a feeling that the differences for us will be even more keenly felt.

The arrival of our next child will definitely be a new adventure and one that I welcome wholeheartedly, with all the ups and downs that may accompany the journey. I am so happy to have another child to love, and I am so excited that Benjamin will have a sibling to grow up with. I look forward to watching their relationship unfold. I am eagerly anticipating Italy, but I will continue to cherish Holland!

Step by Step

We have waited over three and a half years for this milestone, and at the time of this writing it is not yet fully achieved. When I learned that I was pregnant with our second child, one of my initial concerns was, "How can we possibly get Benjamin walking before the baby is born?" I addressed this concern with Rebecca, and she assured me that this would be our main focus in therapy throughout my pregnancy. The issue of walking became a regular prayer request in our home as well because, naturally speaking, it looked so unlikely that Benjamin would reach this milestone any time soon. He was very content to crawl everywhere, and he was still resistant to being held in a standing position, though he was getting into the habit of pulling to stand on furniture *when it was his idea*. I also had a growing concern about lifting him, especially since I had some complications with a low-lying placenta arise at the end of my first trimester. Thankfully, though, that issue resolved itself within the next few months.

In August 2012 Benjamin began attending a school program two mornings a week that is specifically designed for three-year-olds with developmental delays. It is held at one of the local elementary schools, and besides classroom activities, he receives on-site therapy with the school's physical therapist, speech therapist and occupational therapist. He adjusted well to the program, and Shawn and I were so relieved that he would be receiving additional intervention to help him with his development. The weekly in-home therapy we received through Sooner Start had ended in May when Benjamin turned three. A month into the school year, though, I realized that he needed more than just four hours a week of interaction with other children. In the weariness of pregnancy, I realized that I needed more breaks as well. So, I looked into the local Head Start child care program and began the process to get him enrolled. I attended Head Start as a child and had a positive experience, so I was optimistic about taking this route. Shawn and I thought it would be very good for our son to be around a larger group of typically-developing children. The agency was willing to tailor things for Benjamin's unique situation and allowed me to sign him up for only two mornings a week. They also assured me that an aid would be provided for him to assist with his specific care needs. He was able to start the program near the end of October, and after a rocky first few days, he got settled in and now loves to go! He has been blessed with an amazing teacher and wonderful aid, who he absolutely adores. Our son is now receiving intervention and reinforcement of the things we are working on from multiple sources!

We continued to work hard in physical therapy. Our biggest hurdle was figuring out how to teach Benjamin the concept of placing one foot in front of the other to take steps. He was cruising the furniture stepping side to side by this point, though he had a tendency to drag one leg behind the other. One day in therapy Rebecca and I both sat down feeling perplexed by this issue. After the progress we had been making, it felt like we had hit another wall that Benjamin was presently unwilling to scale. We had tried so many different things to motivate him to take forward steps, all to no avail. In one final attempt, she had me sit on a stool several feet away and start encouraging Benjamin to come to me. The next minute, we suddenly had a breakthrough! Benjamin is still very much a Mommy's boy, and even though he is with me most of the time, this became the motivation he needed to move his feet forward with her assistance. We were both ecstatic as he smiled and laughed and moved in my direction! In that brief moment, something flipped in his brain, and Benjamin grasped the concept of stepping forward instead of side-to-side. I call it Divine intervention!

With this large hurdle behind us, we were now ready to introduce Benjamin to a child-size walker that was designed to be pulled from behind. Rebecca pulled one out soon after and had Benjamin practice standing with it while holding the handles. He wasn't sure what to think of this new contraption, and, as usual, he was resistant to the change. However, it didn't take long before he started to grasp the concept of how to use the walker to his advantage. Shawn and I were amazed at how quickly he took to this new-found skill. Before long he had learned to pick up speed and to re-adjust himself when he bumped into something. Shawn started taking him on walks around the block, and though it was often slow-going, Benjamin loved every minute! He was experiencing a new level of independence, and his strength and stamina were increasing. Meanwhile, we continued to work on having him walk with our assistance. We practiced at home almost daily. I would sit on one side of the living room with his favorite toy (a See-and-Say) in hand and spin it while Shawn supported him at the other end of the room and helped him move towards me. Bit by bit, he required less support as he began to gain his confidence. Sometimes our little guy would hold his own hand as he took shaky steps towards me. Though I'm not sure that it helped him physically, he definitely found a level of psychological support using that method! I was so relieved that I could now hold Benjamin's hands and walk him places, since he had become too heavy for me to carry around.

Over the Christmas holiday break, Rebecca encouraged us to take the walker to the mall for practice. It wasn't until we arrived that I realized we had never had our son use his walker in this large of a public setting before. Shawn had already considered that fact and was feeling a little apprehensive. Within moments we were very much aware of the stares from passers-by. However, we took things in stride and encouraged our son along. Meanwhile, Benjamin was having a great time! We were shocked and thrilled that he was able to go the entire distance around the little mall. We had to laugh inside by the end of the outing. A three-year-old with a walker is not a sight you see every day, much less a three-year-old who is as enthusiastic as our little boy behaved. He let out shouts and squeals of delight *the whole time.* We really couldn't blame people for looking, and we were so proud of him!

By the beginning of the New Year, it was becoming obvious that Benjamin's season with the walker would be a short one. In fact, we just retired it for good on February 3! The month prior, on January 8, there was much rejoicing when my little boy took independent steps towards me during his physical therapy appointment! Shawn was thrilled to hear the news, and we were able to get him to take some more independent steps during our practice times at home over the next week. January 14 was another magical day for us. When I picked up my son from Head Start, his teacher told me that he had taken 6-7 steps on his own initiative! I couldn't wait to tell Shawn when he got home! Benjamin and I were playing with a toy at the end of our living room nearest to the front door when my husband walked in. I immediately told him the good news and then stood Benjamin up and encouraged him, "Walk to Daddy!" With a huge grin on his face, our little boy took 7-8 steps all by himself into Daddy's waiting arms. It was the first time he had ever walked to Shawn before. A very proud father enthusiastically exclaimed, "Yay! You walked to Daddy!" Then with tears in his eyes he repeated, "You walked to Daddy." I started to cry too. There are no words to express the joy and gratitude that rose up in both of our hearts at that moment. We had waited and waited and waited for this, and it was overwhelming and a bit surreal that it was finally happening.

Less than a month has passed since that milestone at the time of this writing, and our little champ continues to make progress. He's still not walking independently on a regular basis, but we know it won't be long. As we eagerly anticipate the arrival of our beautiful daughter Joelle at the end of this month, I am filled with gratitude as I look back and consider how far Benjamin has come over these last several months. What felt so impossible has become a reality. Our prayers have been answered, and all the hard work has paid off as we keep taking things step by step!

No More Excuses!

Where has the time gone? During this last year of pregnancy and welcoming our daughter into the world, Benjamin seems to have suddenly grown up before my eyes. A year ago he was still crawling everywhere, pulling to stand with lots of support, and being carried all the time. Though he was three, he was still operating in a baby stage in many ways. Now at age four he is walking all over the place, getting into everything, and able to go from happy laughter to angry temper tantrum and back again in less than a minute! Shawn and I are extremely proud of the progress our son has made this year, but we are also becoming more painfully aware of his current delays and behavior issues. While every child with Down syndrome will develop at their own unique pace, we are realizing that Benjamin could be farther along in several areas had we been more intentional. We had a heart to heart about this recently and reminded each other, "No more excuses!"

As I have clearly communicated already, raising a child with Down syndrome holds many joys and many challenges. There are no easy answers for anything. Intervention is essential for Benjamin to progress in his abilities, and this means extra work, extra frustrations, and extra tears from all parties involved. Since he is not yet verbal, it is often difficult to discern what his level of comprehension is in any given area. It has been very easy to make excuses. It's been easier to play the "Elmo's World" movie than to deal with a temper tantrum. It's been easier to give him more assistance than necessary when he's eating than to clean up the mess he creates on his own. It's been easier to give him the soft spout sippy cup that he chews on than to fight with him to drink from an open cup. It's been easier to let him play with the familiar toys than to deal with the screams and cries when we introduce something new. The list goes on. Now, we don't always take the easy way out, and there have been countless times that we have worked hard with him over extended periods to develop new skills. However, we've realized that with the extra responsibility and demands on our time with a second child we've been more and more prone to let things slide. What's easier in the moment, though, does not serve Benjamin in the long run. No more excuses!

A few years ago a ministry team prayed over Benjamin while we were visiting the International House of Prayer in Kansas City. One person shared with us, "Others will say that he can't do *(fill in the blank)*, but God says he can!" At the time I envisioned the "He can't..." coming from people on the outside. I pictured battles with school officials, medical professionals, or kids from his peer group. However, the morning Shawn and I had our talk, I came to the sobering realization that I have been the guilty party! Even if I haven't actually said that Benjamin can't do something, it's been communicated by my own attitude and actions. I asked the Lord to forgive me and to give me greater vision for my son's life. As I tearfully shared this with Shawn, my sweet son threw his arms around my legs laughing and grinning from ear to ear. He looked up at me with delight in his little face as if to say, "It's OK, Mommy. I love you!"

As I said, there are no easy answers with Benjamin, but we know the One who holds all the answers. We may feel so inadequate in ourselves to face the challenges of raising a child with special needs, but the same God who knit Benjamin together in my womb lives inside of us, and He will supply all the grace we need to raise our son well. When I feel overwhelmed I must ask myself, "Am I accessing that grace?" In those moments it's good to remember what the Lord spoke to my heart during my son's first year:

I have chosen Benjamin for Myself, and I will release My glory through him. His condition is not a tragedy but an opportunity for

Me to show Myself strong. Do not grow weary and do not lose heart for I have chosen your family for such a time as this. I will yet wipe every tear from your eye and restore joy where there has been sorrow. I AM God and I will do this, so look to Me. Always look to Me.

No more excuses!

A Time to Cherish

"One of the best things you can ever do for your son is to have another child." I heard these words during several physical therapy sessions before that happy day in July 2012 when we learned I was finally pregnant for the second time. We had always planned on having more children; having a child with Down syndrome neither discouraged nor motivated our desire. However, I was (and still am) excited about the benefits Benjamin will receive from having a sibling. On the flip side, though, we were also told to expect that new layers of grief would emerge upon the arrival of a "typical" child. Watching our next child naturally develop would cause us to recognize more and more just how hard our son has had to work to meet his developmental milestones.

During the months I was pregnant with Joelle, I was intentional to ask the Lord to speak to me about her life. I remember the day He whispered to my heart, *Enjoy her! Enjoy the process of growth. She will be a healing balm.* As we are now quickly approaching the celebration of her first birthday at the end of next month, I am keenly aware of how true all of the dynamics mentioned above have been—benefits, grief, joy and healing.

The healing began early in the morning of February 28, 2013. The evening before, I cuddled Benjamin next to me on the couch as he drifted off to sleep. It was a bittersweet moment as reality hit that this was the last time it would just be Benjamin and Mommy. Starting the next day he would have to share me. I held him close and soaked in the memory we were creating. I could barely sleep that night, due in part to the discomforts of late term pregnancy, but even more so because of the anticipation of knowing we would soon meet our baby girl! When the alarm went off before the crack of dawn, I was eager to change into my comfy fleece pants and pull-over and head for the hospital. My mom, who had arrived the week before to help with the new baby, sleepily saw us out the door. "Dana, you're glowing!" she exclaimed.

Shawn and I talked and prayed as we made the drive across town. It was such a new feeling to know we were having our baby today in contrast to the shock of Benjamin's early delivery nearly four years before. As the surgical team began to prep me for the C-section, I prayed that Jesus would hold me and surround me with His peace, for I clearly remembered the terror of my previous experience. While the spinal was being administered, a calmness rested on my heart, and I knew this time it was going to be so different. Soon my newborn daughter's shrill, strong cries pierced the air, and I smiled confidently that she would have no difficulty breathing on her own. It was hard to contain my excitement as she was cleaned, weighed and measured. I was going see my baby right away this time! My heart felt like it would burst when Shawn held our swaddled daughter by my head so I could look at her and kiss her face while my surgery was being completed.

Once in my hospital room I had only a short wait before little Joelle was placed in my arms. My mom walked into the room less than a minute later, her face beaming, as I serenely said, "I just got her!" It was a beautiful moment. There were no tubes, wires or ventilator to hinder my view of her tiny features. Instead of touching little hands and feet in a NICU bed, I had my baby where she belonged—cradled in my arms, close to my breast. It was a very healing day!

I won't go into all the details about the contrasts that accompanied the next several weeks as Shawn and I had the first time experience of caring for a healthy newborn. Joelle was a high-maintenance baby from day one, and we were exhausted! While I was pregnant, all I could think about was how glorious it would be to bring a healthy baby home right away. I was so thankful that she was healthy and that she was home, but I had underestimated the degree of work and energy that would be involved, especially while recovering from major surgery. I used to have to wake Benjamin up to nurse. Now I was praying that my baby would sleep for just a little bit between feedings! It took a while before we got into a rhythm and life began to have a normal balance to it again.

During these last ten and half months, I feel like I've had to learn to be a parent all over again. I know that every child is different, but I believe that when you have a child with a disability the differences are so much more apparent. It has been both thrilling and heart-wrenching at times to watch Joelle's natural progression of development. As she will suddenly master a new skill, I will remember the great amount of time and effort involved for Benjamin to reach the same milestone. The day I first offered her a sippy cup I was shocked as she immediately latched on and began to suck. I have been amazed at her alertness and curiosity as well as her motor and language development. Last week I was reading a book to her and pointed at a picture on the page. Without skipping a beat, she extended her index finger and pointed at every page in the book as we continued to read. I wasn't trying to teach her to point; she just did it. I was a bit dumbfounded because one of the skills Benjamin's speech therapist and we are currently working on is to teach him to point!

With speech in mind, there was the amazing day when Joelle was eight months old, and she spoke her first purposeful word. She was sitting in her high chair while Shawn, my mom and I were seated around the table. (Grandma Jan had just recently moved from across the country to the house across the street!) Looking at me, Joelle began to say, "Mama! Mama!" and clearly wanted me to hold her. It was one of the most beautiful moments of my life as a mother. I had waited over four years to hear that word spoken to me! My heart melted to hear it from my baby girl, but there is grief that I am still waiting to hear it from my son. I know it will come in time, just as so many other things have before.

Though they are nearly four years apart, many of my interactions with Benjamin and Joelle are very similar at this point. The same games and songs bring delighted squeals and laughter from both. The same books and movies capture their attention. The same toys are played with (and fought over). There are moments when I want to laugh and cry, such as the day when both children sat on the floor chewing on a sock! In those moments, I have to choose to laugh. In those moments I have to remind myself to enjoy and cherish the present. The developmental stages that have felt so dragged out with Benjamin will continue to progress over time, and I don't want to look back with regret that I didn't savor this time when my children are young.

I also have to remind myself how very far my son has come since the arrival of his sister. I remember so well the day I was still recovering in the hospital, and Shawn brought Benjamin in to see me with the news that he had just walked unassisted all the way from the parking garage! It was a huge turning point and answer to prayer. He is now walking around everywhere and gaining greater independence. He is learning to feed himself and play with more focused attention. He is communicating through some sign language, and is thrilled to attend Pre-K every morning. He is branching out to new relationships and becoming more and more of his own little person. I am so proud of him!

As anticipated, the adjustment to having a sibling has been a challenging one for Benjamin, but overall he has handled the change better than we expected. His initial response when we brought Joelle home from the hospital was to ignore her. (He even ignored me for the first day, which I never would have imagined)!

In time his curiosity won over, and he began to look at her and touch her, often smiling and laughing as he did so. For the most part he has been gentle with her, though there has been some hitting along the way. He is also careful to step around her when she's playing on the floor. There is definitely jealousy, too, as he adjusts to sharing Mommy and Daddy's attention, not to mention his toys! However, none of his responses have been any different from what would be expected from any first child. Joelle continues to be fascinated by her big brother and everything he does. She is so eager to follow him and try to do whatever he's doing. This will really get interesting once she begins walking! I look forward to witnessing the continual unfolding of their relationship.

The contrasts between my two beautiful children will become more and more apparent as time goes by, but I am reminded that I need to celebrate them both at exactly where they are and for who they are. Even as I drove to the coffee shop this morning with this reflection already composing itself in my mind, I found myself praying, "Lord, help me be free to be me. Help me to be who You intended for me to be." My children remind me that we all have different areas of strength and weakness, and we need each other. We are to bear with each other in our weaknesses and rejoice with each other in our victories. Above all, we are called to love. As I raise my children I want to maintain the perspective that **the greatness of their lives will not be measured by their level of abilities but by their ability to love**. My greatest dream for them both is that they will love Jesus, the Lover of their souls, with all that they are and that they will extend that love to those around them. This will be a life well-lived, a life to be cherished!

Dream Come True

What do you want to be when you grow up? This is a question that children are asked throughout their years of childhood, and their answers may change from year to year (or day to day) as they develop and mature. I remember the many answers I had to this question during my own childhood years: *singer, writer, teacher, actress, veterinarian* (only for a short time until I realized I would actually have to do things that involved blood and needles, not just play with animals all day)! While many things from this list still ring true to the passions of my heart, there is one answer that has always been deeply rooted inside of me, unchanging amid the many changes of childhood, adolescence, and adulthood. *What do you want to be when you grow up?—a* **Mommy***!*

As a teenager I would have told you that my ideal life scenario would be to marry a pastor and be a stay-at-home mom. I envisioned the beauty and romance of being married to a godly man and ministering together, raising adorable and well-behaved children, and being a model homemaker as I spent my days in the bliss of motherhood—reading books, singing songs, baking cookies, making crafts, playing imaginative games, etc…In my mind it was a picture of true contentment, my "happily ever after" if you will.

This was my dream at sixteen. At the time that I write this I am thirty-one, and by most outward appearances I am living my dream. I did marry a wonderful and godly man. In our early years of marriage we were involved in youth ministry together. For the last two years we have been ministering in a pastoral role at IHOP-B. He also has the opportunity to pastor young hearts in his new job as special education teacher at one of our local middle schools. I love him and respect him, proud of the man he is and is becoming. I am privileged to be a stay-at-home mom for our two precious children and believe that in time there will be more to come. I do spend my days reading books, singing songs, rocking babies, cooking meals, keeping house, and the list goes on and on... Yet in the midst of these responsibilities and blessings, I've had to come face to face with the restlessness of my own heart. For one thing, when I was sixteen I didn't take into account the amount of hard work and monotony that actually comes with maintaining a marriage, raising a family, keeping a home, and serving in ministry. I also didn't honestly take into account that no dream fulfilled, no matter how beautiful or noble, can truly satisfy my heart—only Jesus can.

I was talking with my husband in the car awhile back and shared with him some of the struggles I was experiencing. I was feeling lonely in my role as a homemaker. I was feeling disappointed that I am limited in the activities I can be involved in, especially at our church. I was feeling discouraged thinking I was missing the mark in almost every area of my life. I felt like I was somehow "missing out." As is often his advice, Shawn exhorted me to ask the Lord for His perspective on what I was feeling and allow Him to change my paradigm. Somewhere in the midst of this conversation I recognized the irony of my own woes and had to laugh at myself. *You said you wanted to be a pastor's wife and homemaker. God has given you the desires of your heart!*

Recently the Lord has been bringing me wonderful encouragement concerning my role and calling as a mother. Some of it has been through the heartfelt writing of other moms, some has been through spoken testimonies, and some has been through His own whispered words to my heart. *But Jesus said, "Let the little children come to Me, and do not forbid them; for of such is the kingdom of heaven,* (Matthew 19:14). He has been lovingly reminding me of things I've known to be true but have sometimes lost sight of in the midst of the busyness and demands of each day.

Mothers are given the extraordinary responsibility and privilege of raising the next generation of world changers. We are called to nurture, teach, and disciple the little ones who are to inherit the Kingdom of God. Our words and actions are forming our children's earliest framework for how they will view God; we are called to be a representation of His heart! We are entrusted with stewarding, for a season, the lives of the very ones who hold such immense value in His eyes. These are the ones He created, the ones He poured out His blood to redeem, and the ones who have been in His heart for all eternity. Motherhood is a high calling, but it is a calling that must be walked out in the ordinary, mundane, everyday issues of life. It is also a calling that can only be fulfilled as I set my heart to love and worship Jesus in midst of these very things. This is where true life and contentment is found.

We all have different dreams, but the truth is, no matter how big or small a dream may be, no matter how ordinary or extraordinary it appears, a dream in itself is powerless to bring lasting contentment, and it is ultimately meaningless if it is not rooted in relationship with Jesus Christ. There have been many great accomplishments in the eyes of man throughout history that will be forgotten in eternity. Yet there have been many simple, hidden lives, unnoticed by the world around, loving Jesus wholeheartedly and faithfully serving in the situations of everyday life that will be remembered and celebrated in heaven. This gives me great hope and renewed vision for how I want to live my life in this season and every season. When I focus my heart on Jesus in simple love and worship as I sweep Cheerios off the floor multiple times a day, or as I change another dirty diaper, or as I sing "The Wheels on the Bus" for what seems like the hundredth time, it is noticed and remembered in heaven. When motivated by love for Him no task is insignificant, and it carries the promise of eternal reward. As I speak words of life and destiny into my children and shower them with love and affection as we walk through our very natural days, I am helping to paint a portrait for them of a supernatural God Who loves them immensely and has called them to be His own.

Yes, being a wife and mother is a dream that's come true for me, but the greatest dream of my heart is to be a whole-hearted lover of my Lord and Savior Jesus Christ, to grow in the knowledge of Him, and to represent Him in this world, living as He lived and loving as He loved. It is only in the pursuit of this dream that I can be the wife and mother He has called me to be. This is the dream that must consume all other dreams. This is my true dream of happily ever after!

ABOUT THE AUTHOR

Dana grew up in the Midwest, born in Missouri and raised in Kansas. At age 18 she moved to Bartlesville, Oklahoma to attend Oklahoma Wesleyan University where she studied behavioral science. Her interests during her school years included music, acting, and writing. She graduated from OWU in 2004 and married her best friend, Shawn, at the end of 2005. After spending four years working in the behavioral health field and Christian education, Dana was eager to take on the role of stay-at-home mom upon the birth of their first child, Benjamin, in 2009. Their daughter Joelle arrived in 2013. Shawn and Dana have been on the pastoral team of a small church plant named The International House of Prayer-Bartlesville since 2011. Dana continues to express her creativity through writing, song, and motherhood.

Contact Information: reflectionsfromholland@gmail.com

Made in the USA
San Bernardino, CA
12 September 2014